SHATTERED

Recovering From A Traumatic Injury

Marc Maislen

New Visions Arts Publishing
Shattered: Recovering From a Traumatic Injury

For information contact: newvisionsarts@gmail.com.

The author of this book does not dispense medical advice or prescribe
the use of any technique as a form of treatment for physical, emotional,
or medical problems without the advice of a physician, either directly or
indirectly. The intent of the author is only to offer information of a
general nature to help you in your quest for physical, emotional and
spiritual growth and well-being. To wit, the author and publisher assume
no responsibility for your actions.

Printed in the United States of America.

ISBN:978-1-7364125-0-3 (paperback)
978-1-7364125-1-0 (hardcover)
978-1-7364125-2-7 (eBook)

1. Maislen, Marc 1951-
Editor: Meredith Maislen
Cover Design: Mary Eastman

WITH DEEPEST GRATITUDE TO

Mary Eastman, for her unwavering dedication and understanding. And for truly being there.

SPECIAL THANKS TO

Meredith Maislen, for her tireless work in editing this book.

THANKS TO

The people who read portions of this book and continually encouraged me when I felt like putting the manuscript in a drawer: Bryan Baisinger, David Belmont, Deanne Dunlap, Bobby Faust, Jean Henchman, Morgan Locklear, Cat Mair, Sandy Maislen, Ramon Maislen, Rose Reed, Marian Sandmaier, Rick Silberman and Gloria Weiner.

To the team of professionals, legal and medical, friends and family, as well as others with disabilities who inspired me with their dedication and hard work. Al Laub, Diana Simo, Karen Koehler, Anne Roberson, John and Amy, EMT Northgate Rescue, Detective Bacon, SPD, Dr. Richard Bransford, Dr. Erik Kubiak, Dr. Chip Route, Dr. Douglas Hanel, Dr. Weiyi Ding, Dr. Evan Cantini, Dr. Joseph Wu, Carolyn G. Rodenberg MA, Dr. Laura Beck, Dr. Jeffrey Suver, Shirley Giles RN, Dr. Peebles, Bill Torvund, Susan Palmer, Wayne Saito LPT, Martha Stanton LPT, Linda Hagemeyer OT, Mac Vujovich, Mary & Dave at rehab, Paul J. Curtis, all of my children, Diane Rose, Maggi Murphy, Joan Busto, Michelle Maislen, Fabien Pichard, everyone at the Kline Galland Home, JFS and Jeanne Rose Roxby.

TABLE OF CONTENTS

PART III
DOING THE WORK

PART IV
COMING INTO THE LIGHT

SHATTERED

INTRODUCTION

Tuesday morning, October 6, 2006 was surprisingly sunny in Seattle. What's more, things were going pretty well for me and, like most people, I was living my routine. Reflecting back, I was a married 55 year old man with five grown children. The description, "prime of his life" is certainly subjective but, that's how I felt. I was healthy and still very much interested in exploring life which had both a conventional and unconventional side to it.

After settling in Seattle in 1999 and taking a break from art, I became director of a K-8 school. And as my planetary awareness and social consciousness gained traction, I shifted gears and became the major gifts officer for a company called Climate Solutions which was dedicated to fighting global warming. My origins were on the East Coast where the unconventional part of me had been a professional dancer and an American Mime. I also had my own theatre/dance company, producing and performing original works in New York City and Boston. As luck and life would have it, I eventually decided to shift gears and move West to perform and direct theatre. As a movement/theatre artist I relied on my body to respond instantly to thoughts and emotions in order to theatrically express myself and prior to October 6th I was a Certified Personal Trainer (ACE) and Spin Instructor. In short, all was going well...

Upon reflection, on this day I was heading southbound to work in downtown Seattle on Aurora Avenue. That was my intention anyway, until the unpredictability of life intervened. Even though I was doing "good work," a strange complacency was beginning to dominate me. Not the kind of sitting around doing nothing couch potato complacency, but the sneaky kind. The kind where the worm nibbles away at the sweet core of yourself without taking large pieces; without disturbing you enough to make you aware that the center is being eroded bite by bite. It was this complacency, like the tides awash over me, which caught me in the undertow. While having many accomplishments and a diverse life, there was a sense of incompletion prior to the collision that I couldn't put my finger on.

As I left my house I briefly stopped my car in front, scampered up the five steps and grabbed a water bottle from my wife before giving her a kiss goodbye. I had no inkling that my quick pit stop would set the wheels in motion that would end my days of playing tennis and rock climbing forever.

I know I got into my car with my gym bag. I know I headed off to my job raising money to fight global warming. I know I had the usual scenarios floating through my head about life, family and the things I needed to do when I arrived at the office. I could not stop the nagging feeling that I had not yet achieved what I wanted in my life. I felt I was becoming invisible. I feared I might vanish. I always believed the value we attributed to life's milestones is evaluated through a discerning eye tempered by sweet experience but because of amnesia I still don't remember what happened on Aurora Avenue that morning.

Nevertheless, I am forever touched by the story of the woman in the car next to me. She was in the car to my left when the truck crossed the road. She smashed her brakes while swerving her car to the left and barely cleared the rear of the truck as she heard the impact of my car colliding underneath the semi. She was so shaken up she was unable to continue driving and immediately pulled over to the side of the road where she proceeded to weep uncontrollably. What was revealed to me later was that her infant child was in the car with her and she wept both in fear and gratitude for the life of her child. That was where the police found her to record her statement. Only after calming down was she able to continue driving. Here was both the tragedy of my crash, being run over by a truck driver who was high on drugs while driving a 20,000 pound semi-truck, and the miracle of her and her child's survival living side by side.

So here I am in my car on the way to work when I am thrust into a totally new chapter of a different book than the one I lived, rehearsed and thought I knew. My memories are flashes and pictures at this point; fuzzy but violent – I am being rushed into surgery - my arm bone sticking out of my skin. Shattered pieces of elbow and hip must be reconstructed if I am to use my arm or leg again. Are these actually my recollections or a script which I somehow pieced together from what I was told well after the fact? The police came to the ER to check whether my injuries would be fatal so they could decide what charges to file against the driver of the truck. Somehow I lived through this although half of the top of my small Ford Escort had been crumpled and ripped off over my head. I am lucky the truck did not act as a guillotine. I survived.

That morning when I loaded my gym bag into my car and headed to work, I never imagined that within ten minutes I would lay trapped in my car, pinned under the middle of a semi-truck that had crossed the highway directly into my path, dragging me fifteen feet until the transaxle of the truck broke, stopping its progress. I never imagined that ten minutes after kissing my wife goodbye, I would have broken bones protruding from my body, a cracked femur exploding my hip socket into pieces and my skull ripped open by glass and metal. I never imagined that instead of spending the day working to raise money for global warming and then teaching a Spin class, I would be cut out of my car by the Jaws of Life® and rushed into emergency surgery for the next seven and a half hours, followed by two more surgeries of almost equal duration to repair my damaged body.

As I dance between recollections, reconstruction of facts and my true memories, I can see in my mind's eye a peach sunset with light indigo trim. I visualize a more innocent time in my teens where the glimmer of the sun is winking at the sky's beauty, like the peek from the girl in the second row as she turns to make eye contact with me. Through it all, I can still feel the skipping child inside me, leaving a trail of fall leaves in his wake. As they swirl in the soft breeze I am imagining the contrail of a jumbo jet behind me, my feet no longer touching the ground.

This is about me soaring into the unknown.

When I alight again four years later in 2010, I cannot walk more than a few blocks at a time and I only have limited use of my right arm, but I understand that I am not destined for complacency. I still on occasion wake my wife because I am moaning in my sleep but I have found the humor and lightness of being, without being sarcastic or acid. My laughter is full and rich and unashamedly deep.

What you will read in the following pages is not about winning a gold medal at the Olympics. Rather, this is a mosaic of loss, sadness, wonder and discovery. It is about an unexpected journey. More importantly, it is about shining a light on the shadow of pain; my pain. It is about washing the pain away, enabling me to begin walking the path of recovery; my recovery. As I look back on the cataclysm of events that nearly brought my life to an end, I have realized that, in one sense at least, it pushed me to the razor's edge of choice where I was permitted to look closely at the unfolding unique map of healing. From here I would experience a greater appreciation of life; my life.

Your map and my map will be different. My hope is that you can use the experiences I relate in this book as a stepping stone for yourself to break through the barriers which may have prevented you from retrieving some of the things you have lost and inspire you to live the life you long for.

Shattered

5

Man hurt in Aurora Ave. crash

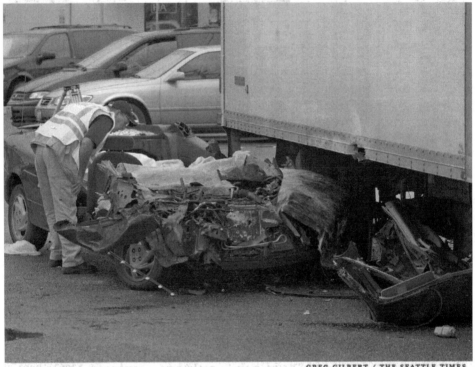

GREG GILBERT / THE SEATTLE TIMES

A member of the Seattle police traffic-collision-investigation squad inspects a Ford ZX2 car that ended up partially under a large truck after a collision Friday morning on Aurora Avenue North near North 107th Street. The crash happened about 9:30 a.m. The car's driver, a 55-year-old man, had to be cut out of his vehicle, and he was taken to Harborview Medical Center with serious internal injuries, police said. The truck driver, a 24-year-old man, was not injured.

PART I
ENTERING THE DARKNESS

Chapter One

OVERVIEW

PTSD recollection from my car right after impact:

"Blood being wiped from my face. I am able to see my arm as my blood is seeping through my jacket. Unrelenting pain. Trapped and unable to move, my breath shortens. I need air. Please give me air. I cannot breathe. Oh God, I need air. Air."

As an active healthy man I never dwelt very long on the subject of injury, pain and recovery. But after having a traumatic injury it became clear to me that people have little understanding of what the injured are going through, any more than we ourselves do. Although each one of us is an individual experiencing whatever life has brought to us, after severe trauma to the body, all this changes. After years of building a reality and having that reality drastically altered, sometimes in a moment, the world view of who we are is suddenly not understood, either by ourselves or by others.

I discovered just how true it is that life takes on a richer meaning after one has a near-death or catastrophic experience. Isn't it strange that we are oblivious to our parents and teachers when they tell us how fragile, brief and vital life is? Clearly we are. Why else would we need to experience tragedy in order to produce dramatic gains?

We have all noticed how people generally progress through life: growing up, getting married, having kids, securing jobs, changing jobs, possibly re-marrying, getting old and dying. This progression is not much of a risk when viewed in terms of a rollercoaster ride and indeed, this example demonstrates the safety of going gently around on the carousel of life. Most would agree this is a stable and satisfying path. There is comfort in knowing we can pay the rent or feed our family. As daily challenges are presented we overcome them in understandable, acceptable terms.

It is obvious how comforting this may be for most people, but for those of us who have sustained a life-changing injury there is no comfort. The devastating event has fundamentally changed our lives; its tone, pacing, attitude and sense of future. How shocking is it that something has happened shattering our normal, ongoing picture of the world, forcibly shifting our lives onto an alien and unrecognizable track. Most of us have spent the greater part of our lives on firm ground but, in a single, shocking moment we have been thrust into a totally unfamiliar existence.

Even though I had seen movies with violent car crashes and watched the evening news depicting massive collisions, nothing could have prepared me for the level of pure agony and uncertainty I was experiencing.

I was living an ordinary life with reasonable expectations, so the pain of a crushed, broken body did not figure into my equation. Why would I imagine such a circumstance? Most of us live a routine life; reality easing into a manageable existence. Like settling into your favorite chair, relaxing in its cozy embrace, there is inherent security in going to work to bring home a paycheck. This feeling of comfort more than makes up for the wildness of hitching through Europe while living out of a backpack with wanderlust.

Over a very short period of time I realized that virtually everyone I knew continued to live in the secure world I had just exited. People did not have a true understanding of what I was going through; nor did I wish it upon them. While there was an enormous outreach of attention and compassion from friends, family and professionals, the overarching truth was that I was experiencing this damage, this constant and debilitating pain, this isolation, alone. It was my challenge…a challenge

I must truly face alone.

When I realized that what I was suffering through was not a dream I began to feel a profound sense of loneliness. After having normal contact with friends and acquaintances on a daily basis, there was a gaping hole where social connectivity previously existed. I felt as if I had fallen into a great abyss and no matter how much I yelled no one could hear me. My damaged, incapable self not only felt terribly vulnerable but I also felt that no one else could understand what I was going through. My world was reduced to a bed and the limited area of my house. What if nothing ever changed; if my condition was permanent? What if my bed and house became the extent of my world? I wasn't just alone, I was afraid. In fact, I had never been more afraid in my entire life.

There are many qualities that make us unique, distinguishing us from our friends, conferring our individuality upon us. For example, I enjoy having distinctive curly hair and a toothy smile. But suddenly it became apparent that bodily damage and the commensurate pain was a new defining point in my life. I was also forced to realize this unexpected uniqueness, as defined by damage and pain did not bring me closer to others and was not a socially acceptable reality. After all, we are taught that other peoples' aberrations are "their" issue and "their" problem, not ours. Now I was one of "them" and it was scary that I was not in control. Whether I liked it or not, this isolating experience and condition forced me to examine myself, my attitudes and my motivations, and then summon courage I never thought I had in me.

It is far easier being brave when one is in a crowd. I remember being tear-gassed during the protests in the 60's and feeling so cool being a part of the action. But when a gang of teenagers mugged me in New York City I did not feel so big or strong. Now, when I am alone with my injuries, like being helpless at the whim of the gang, I am riddled with fear. In fact, I was feeling so insecure and "less than" in my new state that I thought it would take a miracle to ever be whole again. It had not yet occurred to me to be thankful for the miracle of survival. I felt like I had hiked high into the wooded mountains without a compass and having been turned around, could no longer find a way out. It felt frightening to speculate that perhaps I would never stop being turned around; being permanently lost. At this stage of recovery it is not clear what being brave means.

There were no easy answers for me in dealing with pain and recovery. The dominating and difficult realizations were that I needed to continually participate in a process that was not only extremely uncomfortable but also did not have a clear and defined end point or outcome. Every day brought new twists, turns and tests for me to tackle.

At times I felt as if I was sitting in a sauna; the sweat dripping the very life blood out of me. Was I going to shrivel up into a prune, then a raisin and finally disappear? Or would I slowly sip the soothing water and incrementally refresh myself? I hoped that once I was wrung out I could fill myself with new building blocks and grow stronger. At other times it was as if dreams were pulled from my memory, allowing me to vicariously relive those parts of my life which have become distant.

As days stretched into months and years I understood it was specifically through this life-changing event that I was able to discover a deeper truth within myself. But to uncover and cast light upon this deeper truth I needed the strength produced by gathering my resources together.

My memory supplies me with images and feelings that feed into health by shining light on who I am, the pure center of my self. A personal story comes to mind. I see there is a majestic oak tree in the woods behind my house. The angle of the trunk allows me to shimmy to the lowest branch. While scraping upward, the wizened skin of the oak grates against my exposed forearms and thighs through my weathered jeans. I do not know whether the tree is trying to repulse me or whether the pressured opposition of the bark is like the signature of the oak I must interpret in scaling its heights. It is the Braille I am forced to read, now that I cannot rely on my eyes at this stage of the ascent. It is all about the feel.

In climbing, I cannot see the upper limit of my progress. Just as in recovery, the assumption that a final plateau exists fires the desire to persevere. Mounting the behemoth that is "oak" I am more concerned with my safety rather than the reward of the magnificent vista once at the top. As the branches get thinner, support is riskier and the danger of failure lurks underneath each foothold. Another challenge of courage.

Where there is a warning pressure from the antagonistic bark of the tree, no such signal emanates from the ever-smaller branches forming the oak's canopy. At this stage of progress, the soft branching crotches barely support my hand hold; placing a foot and full body weight edges me toward danger. To plunge downward would wipe out the gains of recovery in one broad stroke. But traversing the oak's path, sensing where support is greatest, and respecting when the oak is denying access is part of my natural intelligence.

Taking in the breathtaking landscape, eyes no longer blind, a glowing heat infuses the leaves and then my skin. How it must have felt high up in the crow's nest scanning the rolling sea for land, for other ships, for whales, or simply to allow the flight of one's imagination. Like an innocent child, I can become a soaring eagle up here. I can collect all my limitations, draw them together and bounce them away, banishing them into eternity here at the edge of the oak.

Just like a dreamscape, no Euclidian geometry exists here; perhaps only a fractal understanding of the topography of my self. Each serrated leaf represents aspects of my growth into wholeness where the sky is not the limit but a microscopic evolution forming a grand design. I am a survivor scrambling through the maze of underbrush to arrive, out of breath at the living, vibrant oaken monolith of hope, my feeling of unbridled positivism infusing my being.

These recollections inspire me but I ask myself what resources I now possess to draw from to stay the course for this difficult journey. As scary and unknown this road is, I know the map for it must be drawn from scratch. This is not a dream of mine or a play I've written in which I choose the ending. When the fabric of my reality was shattered, the rebuilding of my body became a symbol for the redefining of my self. What followed were new doorways seemingly appearing out of nowhere and opening to the idea of alternative endings. Like a play, this gave my life an entirely new meaning in both what I was choosing and what was being presented as a choice. Long gone were the days of following a leisurely learning curve. What was revealed was the steep ascent necessary to facilitate disciplined healing. In the past when I worked with individuals as both a Personal Trainer and as an acting/movement instructor, I never imagined that the knowledge I gathered during the years I had spent becoming a trainer, dancer and actor would be tested under such extreme measures. Making this choice was about harvesting the courage to continue.

The idea of choice, what I wanted to do, where I wanted to live, how to spend my time…those things I recognized as natural extensions of self determination were no longer automatic. What I faced after my traumatic event was that the luxury and ease of "choice" was simply gone. Ease was replaced with either doing the work or giving up. No middle ground. If there was any chance of recovery at all, by necessity, my will and determination had to be focused on fundamental building blocks: how to walk, talk and function. I felt as if I was in the kitchen making a sandwich, stacking a fresh set of values onto my "old" life. The taste and smell of the meat and veggies represented the level of awareness and acceptance of these new values. Putting this meal together became the starting point of my still unfolding "new" life.

Then there is the insecurity of what if the sandwich doesn't taste good? What if I should have used mayo instead of mustard? But having the confidence of a lifetime spent organizing my goals, weeding out unwanted actions and gaining a semblance of stability, these new painful and unwanted sensations made me feel like a baby learning to walk. This dizzying inability and insecurity made me feel the sort of impatience that goes hand in hand with a feeling we've all faced: failure. This was not the state of being I wanted to be experiencing.

Resources:

Fearless: Creating the Courage to Change the Things You Can by Steve Chandler
The Power of Breathing (Self-help and Spiritual series) by Dr. Sukhraj S. Dhillo
A Book of Stress Relief Tips by Kathy Berman
Maps to Ecstasy: The Healing Power of Movement by Gabrielle Roth, John Loudon and Angeles Arrien
It's Your Choice! Decisions That Will Change Your Life by Marjorie McKinnon
The Art of Finding Yourself, At Any Age by Karen Sala

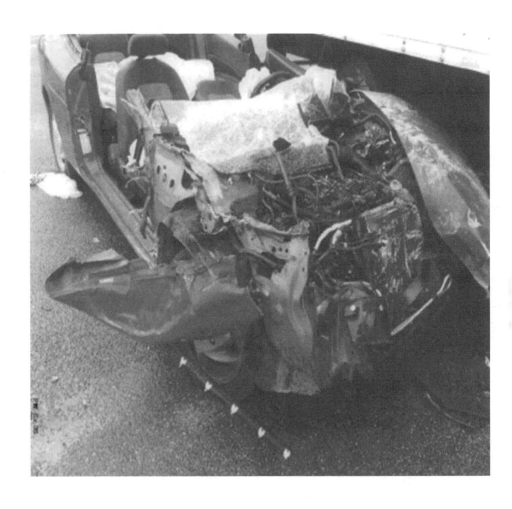

14

Chapter Two

EXPLOSION

PTSD recollection from my Car:

"The noise is deafening. Cutting metal. My teeth chatter uncontrollably. I am cold but it's a sunny Fall day. The noise is surrounding me not as a protection but like spikes sticking into me. Noise and pain. Screaming won't be heard over the sound. Get me out."

Once the collision occurred there was only Emergency Medical intervention in order to save my life. I was not breathing and it was immediately ascertained I had suffered a Traumatic Brain Injury, a 6 on the Glasgow Coma Scale (1=severest, 16=mildest). I was intubated at the scene of the crash.

When all was said and done, I had a compound fracture of my right elbow (a mosaic of bone fragments with my ulna protruding from my arm), a shattered left hip socket (the wall of my hip looking like a broken plate), my right axial nerve severed (result being no longer having the ability to move my deltoid/shoulder muscles), my left femur cracked lengthwise, the left side of my brain suffering from a traumatic brain injury (permanent loss of certain memories as well as speech, word recognition and short-term memory dysfunction), a blood clot in my left leg, and various cuts and abrasions with scarring from glass and metal. Less severe were injuries to my right wrist and both ankles. Later on I also suffered episodes of Post Traumatic Stress Disorder.

A metal rod was inserted into my arm to connect the lower arm to the web of metal now called my elbow. If the non-union fracture (ulna to elbow) did not produce enough bone tissue for the ends to meet, and if bone tissue implanted into my arm didn't produce enough bone, my lower right arm would have to be amputated. My hip was reconstructed with multiple plates and screws recreating the shattered hip wall.

Additionally, due to the hip trauma, half of my Gluteus Minimus (hip flexor) was irreparably damaged and needed to be removed. When it became evident that my axial nerve was destroyed I went through nerve transplant surgery, the thirteenth time it had been done in the world, in which one of the three Triceps nerves was cut and reattached to the axial nerve in the hope of ultimately having deltoid function. Damage to the ulnar nerve produced a lengthy paralysis of my right hand which took about a year to recover from, with residual tingling in my hand present to this day.

Shattered

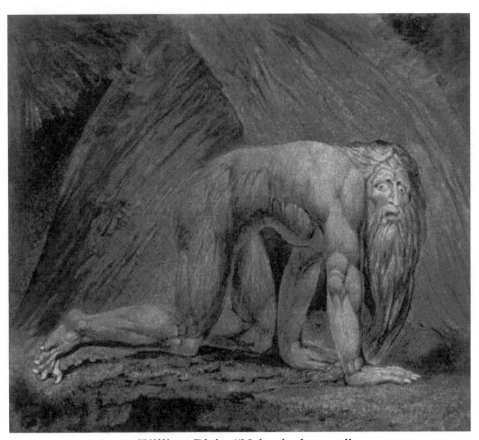

William Blake "Nebuchadnezzar"

Chapter Three

ENTERING THE DARKNESS

My recollection from the Emergency Room:

"I am floating in and out of consciousness. I have no idea where I am. Each time I ask, "where am I?" I am told I am in the emergency room waiting to go into surgery in a few minutes. I don't understand what is being said. I keep repeating myself. I am in agonizing pain. I keep losing consciousness.

When my arm injury, a compound fracture of the right elbow, needs cleansing prior to the surgery the doctors or nurses wash the open wound and protruding bone. I am aware of more agonizing pain and I cannot stop screaming in the pre-op."

My recollection from the ICU:

"I have no memory of the doctors inserting a metal pin through my thigh so that my leg can be in traction prior to surgery to rebuild my hip socket. I cannot roll over in bed or even relax on my side. My left leg must remain immobilized; pulled out by the traction so that the shattered hip socket does not go through any further damage. The wait is three days until the doctors are able to perform the surgery. I repeatedly rise to consciousness asking whether I can move my leg. My oldest son, sister and wife have to calm me down so that I do not move and hurt myself."

Remember entering into your house from bright sunlight? Or climbing up to a pitch black attic? Remember how you don't see anything. When I would imagine what it would be like to cross into the darkness I would think of trying to locate the walls or cleverly use the illumination from my watch to give off enough light to make my way through the blackness. These solutions are not real; they are simplistic, screenplay ideas and do not work in the recognizable world. Standing alone in the dark attic, frozen in how black the darkness actually is, knowing my eyes would eventually adjust, made it acceptable that my racing heartbeat would slow down. But the conception of what is real only existed to the "me" prior to the car crash. Now the blackness was not stopping. It was insidious and frightening.

I understand how darkness can be a protection; being invisible to a threat. Yet darkness, the absence of light, can produce blindness; the inability to see what is happening in the world. Along with blindness comes fear; fear of the unknown. When the boogeyman comes out from the closet or appears unexpectedly from underneath the bed, there is relief and security by drawing the blanket over my head. But what happens when my apparent security under the dark covers is shattered by the bogeyman appearing under the blanket with me?

Once I was devastated by my collision, the conception of the real world also shifted. This shift is the darkness; the uncharted territory of the blinded mind. This new place was inhabited not by my loved ones but by the wandering injured similar to myself. In the darkness I crossed paths with others like myself; others who were as equally alone as I. Having no experience in this "new" world I could not help anyone else because I had no tools to help myself. How long was I supposed to wander in the dark? Would anyone appear as an ally? I was scared.

In my mind's eye I am seeing a world that comes from my imagination yet exists as any reality I have experienced. I close my eyes. I breathe in and out, nice and easy; regular breaths. I see myself before the event. I breathe in the comfort and ease I am experiencing. I exhale my relaxation. All is well. I see the Sun and feel its warmth. I luxuriate in myself. Even with my eyes closed I can "see" the sunlight. Slowly the light is getting dimmer. I don't react much. I keep breathing. Then the dimming light becomes increasingly dark. I squint my eyes open and above me the Sun is disappearing. I think it could be an eclipse but through the darkness I can still see other people and they are not reacting to the change in light. The darkness gets worse until I can no longer see people or anything around me even with my eyes open. Now my heartbeat is picking up speed. I am getting frantic. I tell my body to get up and get out of there but I can't move myself. My panic starts to melt into total fear. Still I can't move. When the blackness totally surrounds me and I feel the pressure of it pushing down on me, I breathe in and relax on the exhale. I see the blank darkness as paint covering a window. I see my hand moving towards the darkness. I feel the sensation that perhaps I will have the ability to slowly peel back the blackness and that something new will be revealed.

As I wonder how I came to this place I had to question whether I willingly stepped over the threshold into the darkness or has entering this dark place been forced on me by someone or something outside myself? Would any of us entertain the thought that we ourselves actually made the choice to finish the life we knew? Prior to my collision the act of voluntarily stepping into the darkness was highly doubtful. Now I had to reconsider this idea.

For example, I know it is a choice whether I choose to eat chicken or roast beef for dinner. That choice is obvious because it is between two things I can see and touch; objects that are tangible. But what if the choice was subtle, even hidden to my everyday eyes? What if the choice was about which direction my life would take and what if that choice was deeply embedded in my subconscious? Would that subconscious choice be any different than the conscious choice of eating chicken over roast beef? It is not. As unbelievable as it seems, I now know that placing my car under a truck and stepping into the darkness is precisely the choice I made.

Years ago I remember being rejected at an audition. My gut wrenching feeling was that the director did not "get" what I was aiming for. My next series of disappointing auditions produced the same result because in my mind it was the directors' fault in their perception of me. Only when a kind casting director pulled me aside to tell me that I kept looking down in her scene did I understand that my failures had nothing to do with the people conducting the auditions. It had to do with me. Transmuting my response of blaming others into "what responsible choices could I make to improve my product" shifted my reality.

When I look at how my life was unfolding prior to my collision, I find I had not yet consciously devised a strategy to develop compassion, patience and humanism. My nagging feelings that life lacked meaning and that I was becoming invisible were somehow tied into this. Something needed to change for me to achieve this growth; and it did. My subconscious designed a plan although I never imagined that the choice I made would take the form of a collision which nearly killed me.

Entering the dark place is indeed scary, unknown, and what would initially appear as a crazy option. Rather than dwell on the 'why would I be so stupid to choose this' it became evident that if I agreed to explore this unfamiliar path and not resist it, I would continue to grow and develop as a person. If I was fortunate I would also become strong enough and sufficiently healthy to reinsert myself back into the world I remembered, albeit in a new way.

Darkness is not simply unconsciousness. Darkness is not a smooth black surface. Darkness is not devoid of life activity. The aspect of darkness that makes it so insidious is that it is alive, can expand or shrink, and can be overwhelmingly thick and bleak. What I felt was that in the absence of my conscious (awake) attention, darkness could ultimately overshadow and dominate my view and blind me to what I needed in order to regain health. This was an enormous revelation.

The pervasive nature of darkness, despair and pain is such that when I was more stable physically, had less agonizing pain, could understand the possibility of growing stronger and was able to recognize the helpfulness of various professionals, the dark shadow had already colored my life and permanently changed me. I would never again be who I was before the collision.

Once again, my subconscious vision/dream approaches reality in my state of recovery. In the black room and before my hand reaches the blackness to peel away the covering, something, some shape emerges from the gloom. Even through total darkness, I can see this shadow figure looming over me, lurking in my vision. This living blackness cannot be avoided. But behind the shadow is a glimmer of light. Not enough for me to see clearly, but bright enough to be hopeful. I gently endeavor to see around the presence of blackness. I breathe in and I have more strength. I breathe in and find myself sliding into the looming black presence. I breathe in and out as I ever so slowly begin to pass through the heart of the darkness.

Piercing through this vision, questions continue to arise. Why did this disastrous event happen to me? Is this a punishment for something I did? Will I ever recover? There is a natural process for this questioning. After all, something did happen to me and I am the one experiencing the after-effects. But I am not the first person to have survived a disaster and I am sure I will not be the last. Through my emotional swings I have not lost the dream of peace and serenity.

Awakening in the morning, the symbolic breaking of the dawn, there exists for me a fleeting moment when the balance of the fresh, sun-warmed morning air combines with the stale yet fresh come-from-dreamland breath. My shift in lung capacity, sleep to awake, deep to shallow is but a reference point to the awakening moment. This fresh, still air resembles the profound quiet experienced in the theatre when an actor, poised and focused, so captivates the entire audience that the air seems to hover, hesitating in pregnant expectancy. To hear a pin drop. For me, everything is possible in that moment.

Unfortunately, unlike the innocent morning wake up, I can only compare my personal awakening in the hospital bed as a twisted, dysfunctional, horror house-like experience. Virtually tied to the bed by multiple tubes, wrappings and casts and further traumatized by the breathing tube filling up my throat, awakening is synonymous with torture.

Each morning was a fresh shock as to what my circumstances had become. I needed to be repeatedly told what was happening so the blackness would not consume my mind. I felt I was on the edge of a precipice with jagged rocks and a dark crashing ocean waiting to devour me.

Fear of the unknown resides as a single point somewhere in my body. In a paranoid delusion, fear furtively moves from one hidden site to another, cloaking its dreadful anxiety and fright in the appearance of normalcy. Terror's recruits gather in battalions awaiting their overlord's command to overrun any semblance of normal life and insert its anarchistic residue into the farthest reaches of my body. Paranoid or not, this is neither a pleasant nor reassuring vision.

When I woke up and got out of bed on the morning of my collision, I had no clue as to what the depth of suffering and pain meant on a daily basis. Neither did I have an awareness of what other people would go through and how their lives and relationships would be fundamentally altered because of my unforeseen catastrophic event.

After my collision, my moments of happiness were abruptly crushed into pain and inability. The feeling of hopelessness was the inky darkness that encroached upon the possibility of small gains to my health. Thankfully, at least at that point, by working with chemical assistance I could short circuit much of the pain. The darkness, however, was much more pervasive.

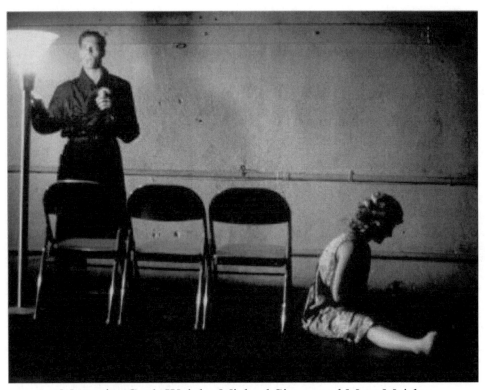
Memories Can't Wait by Michael Simon and Marc Maislen

Chapter Four

WAKING UP

My recollection from the ICU:

"Why am I here? What has happened? What is happening? Each time I slowly ooze through the thick fog that is my consciousness I am awash in confusion. I am lying on my back. I have been intubated since I needed breathing assistance when I was cut out of my car in the street. I cannot focus for more than a few seconds. Thankfully I am not struggling to breathe but I am so sedated that the world makes no sense, has a viscous quality, and is devoid of any relation to ongoing 'time'."

* * * *

"People are like stained-glass windows. They sparkle and shine when the sun is out, but when the darkness sets in, their true beauty is revealed only if there is a light from within."
                    - Elizabeth Kubler-Ross -

I never understood that while peering out my window, whether amidst the incessant hum of the city or in the quiet of rural America, how deeply I was psychically participating in life around me. The sight of wild colored clothes, masses of people and the urban drum beat pounding out rhythms from Tomkins Park filled me with energy. Or the smells of peonies with the background buzz of honeybees producing relaxation within the wash of nature. In both realms I felt the subtle configuration and interplay of internal and exterior worlds. The dance of life.

When the aftermath of my car crash thrust me into isolation with my brain functioning in survival mode and the world of stimulation reduced to a hospital bed, the focal point of my universe became me. When work, shopping, appointments, TV programs, art and relationships became distant specks on the horizon, washed out like a watercolor painting in perspective's blur, the ultimate egocentricity of only "me" right here right now began to coalesce. This moment is a universe apart from the times I just wanted to be left alone to have some quiet time. Here there is nothing outward. No interactivity. No scheduling dilemmas. Only "me."

My window of perception right here right now no longer reveals the familiarity of the world. How easy it used to be swinging my legs out of bed or reaching up to get a coffee mug. Equally disorienting is that the cues I used to traverse life's obstacles are now hidden in a misty soup. The more I try to remove the fog from the window, the sharper its reflectivity becomes. I can't see through it. I can only see a vague image. I get more feverish using my chamois to wipe away the dull coating from the glass, so imagine my surprise when what is revealed is a mirror reflecting only myself. The window to the outside world was no longer transparent.

People act quite individually during life threatening collisions or events. In fact, many people do not lose consciousness. On the other hand, some do lose consciousness and then awaken in a hospital room. My moment of realization, that the room I was in was one I had never seen and was not my bedroom, was my point of awakening.

My waking dream returns with ever more clarity. The wisp of light cutting through the darkness is just enough to calm my fear. Breathing has become regular again as I slowly pass through the inky black figure. Just as I knew the blackness could be peeled back, I know that peeling away the black will show me something surprising. I breathe in and gain courage with each breath. Then I peel away the black and the world on the other side is not one I recognize. There is light. There is space. I feel a sense of relief. The oozy black is not sticking to me. My fear washes away like water running out the sink. I breathe without pressure on my chest. I cast a look past the black and there is a cold, white room. I want to go there even though there is no warmth. I breathe deeply and my sense of relief is being able to shake off the black and make it into the well lit room.

When I awoke in the hospital room, the last thing on my mind was the color of the wallpaper or the quality of the overhead lighting. But like a non-stop camera, my subconscious mind was registering my surroundings. A deep part of my being was aware that this unfamiliar place I found myself in was not my home. But like a punch to the gut, in that deep place I was experiencing fear; fear of the unknown. On the heels of my devastating car crash came a second, albeit more passive devastating event: the hospital.

I don't even like driving by a hospital much less being in one. Yet my rational mind knows that a hospital is a location where we go to get well. But in the initial days after the collision when I was quite medicated, my confused self could not stabilize itself in this radically different environment. Nurses, doctors, and loved ones all talked to me about where I was, that everything was going to be all right. I could not come close to processing that. I could barely discern faces; what was being said made no sense at all. My mind was so overwhelmed I could no more easily accept what they were saying than get out of the bed and go home.

There is more intense light helping to direct me in this fuzzy dream. In fact, I am out of the darkness and into the light. But this light is too bright and my eyes are not comfortable. I blink and blink again hoping my vision clears. I breathe in to steady myself. I breathe in and out and my vision slowly clears. I am no longer moving through space. I see the ceiling. I have no idea where I am. But I know that I am in a room, in a bed looking up. I turn my head and see machines. They are attached to me. I breathe in, in order to stifle a scream. I have gone from black to light. I breathe and look around. I breathe trying to stay calm. I am not sleeping. I am not dreaming. I am awake. An awake nightmare.

Chapter Five

PAIN EXPERIENCE

My recollection from the ICU:

"I am vibrating. Where am I? There is sound. Am I making this sound? I am not thinking clearly. There is so much pain. I know what the sound is. I am moaning. The sound feels like it is being squeezed out of me; the pressure of my body contracting my skin and cells so that I feel like I am being strangled. Like an accordion, my moans are the sad, painful sounds of a broken body exhaling strangely dissonant notes."

* * * *

"Your pain is the breaking of the shell that encloses your understanding."
- Kahlil Gibran –
The Prophet"

Anyone who has experienced constant pain knows it is terribly debilitating. The pain seems to never disappear and firmly wedges itself in, acting as a baseline for all subsequent activities and feelings. Like the drone of a machine relentlessly making background noise, we can sometimes compartmentalize the sound and thereby think that it does not exist. But that is not the case with pain. Pain is much more insidious. Whereas we can tune out sound, pain hurts and cannot simply be disregarded.

I am in the middle of my dream vision again. I am awake. I see the strange room filled with light and machines. Everything is located behind my eyes. I breathe and my eyes relax. There is still a misty confusion as I take in my body. I breathe and see myself. I know something is wrong but I don't know what it is. Slowly another sensation arises. As I connect my mind to my body my heart begins to race. I am experiencing pain. My heart continues to race. The pain is agonizing. The pain is taking over. The mist of confusion is replaced by a fiery blanket with stabbing knives. I have to breathe but every breath brings a ripping sensation to my nerves. This room is like a torture chamber and my body cannot escape. I seem to have awakened into Hell.

Back to the present it is sometimes useful to look at questions visually. So I imagine pain as a curve, specifically a sine wave. Logically the peak of the curve is the high end of pain. If I cut off the top of the curve, forming a plateau, the portion of the curve that has been lopped off most closely represents the removal of the intolerable portion of pain. Luckily, this peak portion of the pain curve is usually limited in duration and so, over time, the agony I initially felt became less severe. As agony diminishes, the next curve of pain arises.

I understand that the critical pain mode is the one where there is a constant, sustained, unrelenting pain whether very intense or more subtle in nature. I understand that the intense pain occurs most frequently at the beginning of the post-event experience and hopefully does not last too long. However, the more subtle pain, the next curve of pain that takes its place, even when quite intense, generally lasts far longer, sometimes years, and is not so easily remedied. Imagine having an ingrown toenail…forever. Not a pleasant thought.

Living with pain is not unique. As crazy as it sounds, desiring pain is not unique either. Many teenage girls who cut themselves with Exacto knives want to feel something; anything to make them feel alive[1]. In their case this is pain. When I looked at my desire to be more complete, to not be invisible, I wondered if there was an aspect of my subconscious that needed to experience pain. Was this the kick start for the engine of the rest of my life? If so, what was fueling this painful creation? I thought my heart desired love, but my eyes, clouded over by my collision could only perceive pain. I needed to rediscover clarity and remove the blinders of limitation. I needed to focus on the dance of life and to find the beat again.

Thankfully, during the collision when my pain reached an intolerable level, I blacked out, protecting myself. I have come to understand that the brain is a tremendously adaptable organ[2]. In my case, I went so far as to be thrown into a state of amnesia where I did not recall the event causing the pain and temporarily forgot the intensity of my pain.

I realized that the gradations of my pain are either quiet reminders of the injuries I sustained or intrusions on every thought and every action

I endeavor to do. When I walk, bend over, grip an object, or when my actions cannot be entered into or completed without the accompanying partner of pain, my daily experience becomes fundamentally different. The activities I once took for granted and what I now observe everyone else doing effortlessly and without thinking are no longer simple and flowing. I must consider the position of my body when doing basic activities. And even with the greatest forethought and care, the underpinning of pain does not go away. It has become the unforgiving truth of my existence. I wonder if I am strong enough to continue to be me. Which begs the question: who is this new person?

Here in the dream/reality I see doctors, nurses and family entering my Hell. But they are treating me with care and kindness and so I realize I am not dead. I breathe and enter back into the darkness. But this is not the same oily blackness as before. I gently and freely enter this darkness as a safe haven from pain. I feel the soothing properties of the pain-killing drugs. I breathe in the relief. A kind of stereo tuner is in front of me. There are knobs for me to turn. I breathe and turn one. The pain gets less. I turn another knob and my vision gets clearer. I rotate another one and my body relaxes. I know I cannot shut out the stereo of pain but I can help tone down the intensity. I breathe in the relief.

I used to go to bed and wake up refreshed and ready to roll. Now there are many days when I awaken from sleep not feeling well. Too often this is a result of a restless evening when subliminal or actual pain is causing me to wake up, on and off, thereby interrupting a full and satisfactory sleep cycle.

The memory of beginning the day bright-eyed and bushy-tailed brings a smile to my face. But beginning the day in pain in no way inspires me to have a positive attitude; quite the opposite. When I start the day in pain with the added overriding condition of being tired, these gray clouds of exhaustion block the Sun, casting a pall over the joy of opening the day with a freshness of spirit. Of course it would be much easier to deny my pain but entering into a state of denial negatively colors so many other aspects of self it is not a wise choice. Stepping into the starting blocks I found it important to first recognize the severity of the pain, the quality of what it is, and whether the pain is causing a blockage of other sensations. I have noticed that generally there is a mix of all three which makes moving through pain and into a more positive, healthy state extremely problematic. But denying my pain is not useful.

There are also days when the severity of pain can be so intense that getting out of the starting blocks to attack items on the to-do list cannot be acted upon. If my hip pain is so sharp that I have to delay or cancel a shopping trip, my normal schedule is affected and my plans need to change. Shifting one's schedule might be easy for most people but my disability highlights my inability to smoothly change gears and reschedule my time. I may not be happy about my difficulty in changing gears, but the elephant in the room casting its shadow is the pain. So the one dominating thought then becomes how can I stop the pain now.

Like a scientist observing and gathering data about a specimen, I examined the pain as if it was alive, having its own identity. Is the pain in my shoulder sharp or achy? Is the pain in my hand only causing stiffness in my fingers or does it radiate up and hinder the movement of my wrist? Does the pain in my hip come and go? Did the pain start when I began to move and go away when I lay down or sat still? Each of these values will determine the next action/response I take in the situation. By being able to examine the pain levels clearly, I give myself a better opportunity to adjust and thereby produce a more positive day to day resolution.

Sometimes when I look down at my hand it feels as if the fingers are crystallizing and sending icy particles into my palm. The sensation is that the blood is conducting irregular electrical charges so that the tingling is separating and dividing reality. I feel as if a Winter storm is brewing as I am struggling across thin ice. The sparkaloid cracking patterns in the ice slowly advance into my body. I am fearful that the tiny fissures will widen and consume me, trapping me in a Winter crystal formation preserving the pain for eternity.

I do not want to be trapped in a pain to pain loop. So I need to ask whether the pain is causing me to disregard or be unaware of the wealth of sensations that are also present at this time. I remember dinners where I missed songs and conversations because the taste of the food I was eating was so overwhelming that it took precedence. The same here. When one sense is over-stimulated, the other senses tend to take a back seat and not be fully experienced. Unfortunately, many of these other sensations taking a back seat are pleasurable. By cutting them off, when I neglect experiencing pleasure, I am eliminating a positive avenue that can be traveled; one that can feed into and assist me in getting through the discomfort of being in pain.

What pleasures can be brought forth and experienced? Something as simple as enjoying the taste of food or listening to George Carlin and laughing can remind me what feeling good feels like. My anchor in the raging sea can be a simple smile.

There is no denying that those of us struck with a traumatic event are experiencing pain with the commensurate degree of pain varying from mild to unbearable. I am not acting like a baby during the times I might be crying or moaning from the intensity of pain I feel. Pain is a signal that there is damage and the body part is not functioning smoothly. I accept that, even through the tears, as I question "why me?"

34

Thankfully, Western medicine is advanced enough to have created a variety of drugs to help diminish pain. Often, taking medication is useful and necessary, however, the nature of the medicine is important to examine.

Opioids attach to proteins called opioid receptors on nerve cells in the brain, spinal cord, gut and other parts of the body. When this happens, the opioids block pain messages sent from the body through the spinal cord to the brain. Opioids affect the way we function and perceive the world because of their interaction with the brain. Because of these functional and perceptual side effects they should be considered the choice of last resort. Other milder solutions such as Advil (ibuprofen) and Tylenol (acetaminophen) can help without altering our ability to control ourselves. Sometimes, taking a couple of Advils or Tylenol can drive the pain level down to a manageable level. This alternative, as a viable mode of treatment, might be examined because these substances are not addictive. Nevertheless, when my pain was agonizing, nothing less than Oxycontin (50-80 mg) would help. Then, after a year and a half, I had to go through the painful process of withdrawal in order to free myself from dependency.

The most important portion of this pain pill dilemma resides in how we place our discomfort; how we identify with it. Obviously, pain is a component of what is happening to us. Also, we alone are experiencing the pain. Given that the experience of pain is personal (our spouse or therapist can only sympathize) it is important to recognize that our experience of the pain is ours alone. So the direction, size and importance placed on the pain are also ours alone. What I am getting at is that we ultimately control the pain by how we choose to experience it.

Have you ever noticed how some people get hysterical and break down when they are injured while others appear strong while in the midst of pain? What creates this?

What I have observed in people who are in pain is that those who are in chronic pain and others who are in the process of shifting from high intensity pain to less pain have something in common: they outwardly display less pain than others who are immediately injured. Why is this? What has changed from the immediate to the long-term? What did the individual do to make the pain manageable?

As I reflect on the idea of an individual taking personal responsibility for the pain he or she is in, it becomes clear. For myself, I know that the pain I continue to experience is not going to go away. Perhaps over time it will disappear but right now it is a part of my daily existence. This "same old same old" awareness has helped me in not having violent reactions to the onset of pain. I don't want to embarrass myself by screaming out in the restaurant because of a sudden shooting pain in my elbow. By placing the pain correctly, it is as if my mind has affirmed the reality of pain and is giving it no more intention and focus than any other feeling. For example, the shock of a loved one suddenly dying would probably cause me to cry uncontrollably with sadness and grief, however, some time later I might cry only when thinking about the loss but not spontaneously and uncontrollably. Am I more insensitive or feeling less than at the onset of the loss? Am I so hardened that I can no longer feel sadness or grief? Not at all. Rather, my perspective has widened and no longer being overly focused on sadness and grief, I can now more fully live my life. Spontaneous crying is no longer appropriate action.

While totally personal in its effect on me, pain no longer dominates and overwhelms me. I experience pain as "just another feeling" I am going through. It hurts, as pain does, but the accent or highlight has been removed.

I have come to realize that it is all about choice. When I wake up in pain I can choose to put an exclamation point on it or I can put a period at the end of the sentence and start a new paragraph, a new thought. This is the miracle of the choice of not identifying who I am with the pain. By making the choice to welcome in all of who I am, not just the "pained one," I am opening myself up to a variety of ways of being without fixating on the pain. Knowing the day might not be an easy one and the pain might not go away is challenging, but observing others successfully handle similar situations I have concluded that moving the pain to the back burner is worth the effort.

I find it remarkable that the administration of pain killing drugs enables the mind to short circuit the connection where the feeling of pain registers in the brain. However, I am not deceived into believing that the pain disappears. There is a constancy of underlying pain and a relentlessness of pain trying to get through the veil of pain killers. Pain has a life of its own; the pain itself is trying to make its presence felt.

The truth is difficult to acknowledge in the early stages of post-trauma; the truth that a degree of pain will be present from this day forward. When I am at a party, having a beer, smiling and cracking jokes, other people looking at me do not recognize that I am in pain. Their minds are wired for feeling and perceiving normalcy. I now live on the other side of the veil where the abnormal constant pain dwells. This is its home and this pain will not disappear.

My dreamscape/reality shows that I at home and feeling at ease in my surroundings. I breathe in, smelling something delicious from the kitchen. I decide to explore. I start to get up and the pain is intense. I try to balance myself but shifting my weight is agonizing. I breathe, body stuck in between movements. My heartbeat is racing. My injury is sucking the strength out of me. I try to deepen my breathing. Breathe. Finally, I am able to sit down again. The pain lingers, sharply knifing into me. I close my eyes and concentrate on exhaling the pain. I breathe in and then exhale the pain. I have some relief. I slowly open my eyes and see the room around me. I am in pain although it has diminished. I am alive. I nod my head in acknowledgment of being alive, happy to have the gift of another day in which to battle through the pain and injury.

Again, examining my progression, my initial step into consciousness and healing was the understanding that I will probably never be pain free. Like when I went off to college and returned home to find my parents had moved. I would never live in the old apartment again. Once I recognized the truth of never being pain free, I was able to embark upon the true healing process. It was vital for me to remember that healing does not necessarily mean that I will be "as good as new" or "back to my old self." Healing is 75% my willingness to be where I am (yes, in pain) combined with the attitude that the experience I have been thrust into is crucial to my growth. This reality is my new healthy state.

Resources:
Dissolving Pain by Les Fehmi and Jim Robbins
The Chronic Pain Management Sourcebook (Lowell House) by David E. Drum

1 Leonard Sax, M.D., Psychology Today, March 14, 2010
2 Kemperman, H.G., et al. (1997), Nature, 386 (6624): 493.
 Manuel Don, PhD, of the House Ear Institute in Los Angeles

Shattered

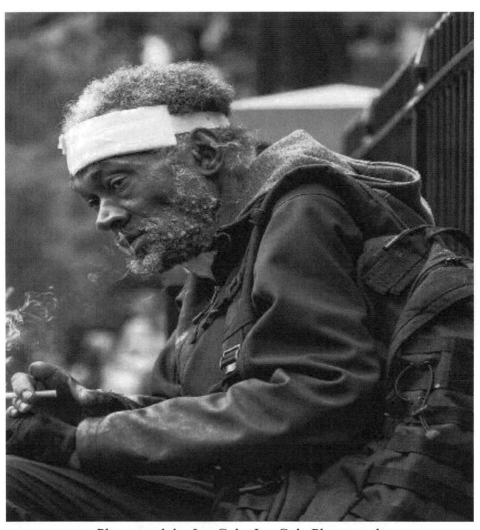

Photograph by Ian Cole, Ian Cole Photography

Chapter Six

WORKING THROUGH IT

My recollection on getting into bed:

"I am exhausted. I just want to sleep. I have to get into bed. I can sit on the edge of the bed but I cannot lean on and use my arm. How am I supposed to get into the bed? I try to use my leg to push up and onto the bed but the leg is so weak and shriveled that I don't have the power to do it. The pain in my hip will not stop. I am left sitting, rocking back and forth, crying. This is not fair. This is not fair."

* * * *

"Never are we nearer the Light than when darkness is deepest."
- Swami Vivekananda -

The pain I was experiencing was the largest deterrent to my progress. In the beginning of recovery, the act of moving caused me enormous pain. At first I was also limited by casts, sutures, and other devices that helped me heal enough before I could begin rehabilitation.

Additionally, pain interrupted my sleep, and without enough rest my recovery was slowed or stopped all together. I cannot recall how many times I was unable to fall asleep or woke up because of pain and could not get back to sleep. I also cannot count how many times I was on the verge of tears (or allowed myself to cry) while asking, "Why me?"

My dream/reality is ever closer to what life is in real time as I experience being brought into physical therapy. I breathe in wondering what is about to happen. I breathe in the activity around me as various therapists are assisting their clients. I look and see many injured people

hard at work. I am worried that I will not be able to do what is required.
I breathe in and out to slow my heartbeat. I breathe in and then exhale a
feeling of ease and relaxation. I am alive. I am dressed. I am not
confined to a room. I am ready and willing to try and work. I breathe in
the fact that this place is part of my new life. I breathe in strength. I am
ready.

Repeating an earlier and ongoing theme, fair has nothing to do with my condition. There is no reason why this event has touched me; it is what it is whether by choice or providence. This oversimplification eliminates superfluous ideas and clears distractions so that facing this new reality becomes part of the process of working it through. Once my tears began to dry up and I awakened to the fact that the pain would not leave me, I started to 'man up'; to do what work was necessary in order for me to become more functional.

I needed to continue taking pain meds for almost a year and a half. In fact, my first rehabilitation specialist insisted that I take pain meds an hour prior to my arrival in the gym because I was making too much noise (grunting) from pain. I eventually throttled my pain response way down; however, each new series of exercises pushed the threshold of my ability to execute them and so renewed my spiking pain. When the body has atrophied, it hurts to get the muscles working. And when there are broken bones coupled with surgery to fix the body, spiking pain is almost always present. Manning up to this pain was a reluctant yet willful choice I made in order to persevere.

I was grateful that my years of dance training ingrained the idea that by employing steady, focused work, incremental changes are inevitable. Progress is the natural product of effort.

Chapter Seven

SUSPENDED

Recollection from the Hospital:

"What is this down my throat? A doctor is about to remove the intubation tube. My insides are coming out. How did this worm get inside me? I am in the movie "The Hidden," throat in spasm choking me. Please stop."

"I am alone with the beating of my heart."
- Lu Chi –

I have said to my kids, "you never know. You could step off the curb and get hit by a car." I never imagined it would happen to me. Yet leaving my house in the morning one day and returning in a wheelchair six weeks later was, as Yogi Berra said, "Déjà vu all over again."

After being discharged from Harborview Medical Center, my world had become the walls of the rehabilitation center. For over a month my activities revolved around multiple sessions with the physical therapist, eating, exercising on my own and at prescribed intervals taking heavy pain medication.

My world circled around strange little "wins." After a week or two I was able to make it to the bathroom unassisted. In rehab when I managed to lift my knee "clam shell style" ten times while lying on my side, my elation was as high as when I received my first paycheck as a performer. I believed at that moment there was nothing I couldn't achieve.

It felt like when I was a kid and had the flu. At that time my world was my bedroom and I thought I would never get out. There was a simple pleasure in drinking ginger ale and the leap to eating a slice of toast was like having birthday cake.

Although the doctors were generally insensitive to my pain since their role was complete, having performed my life saving surgery, they continued to clinically monitor my growing physical strength. In contrast, the physical therapists and nurses were the resident jewels. Like precious stones they were hard on me because they needed to be focused task masters. Yet at the same time, their recognition of each of my gains and the gentleness in which they complimented me were the shining qualities that are so profoundly seen in the facets of beautiful jewels.

When I used to make an entrance onto the stage, the attention from the audience fed me. Just like an audience, the physical therapists listened very attentively to my needs but they translated my needs into a treatment plan, carefully weighing my responses to best facilitate progress. In turn, they communicated with my wife, assuring her of my gains and answering her tough questions. The PTs wholly contributed to trying to make me independent again.

The strangest feeling, however, was mentally structuring every day around the times I could have my pain medication administered. There was a hunger inside me. Like when my wife would slow cook a pork loin and for hours the intoxicating smell would drive and enlarge my appetite. The hunger for the meds was the same. When I would initially take them, the first hour was reasonably pain free and pretty euphoric (opiate drugs are like that). I certainly understood why people abuse them. But as the effects of the drugs from the second through the fourth hour wore off, I became increasingly irritable. My days were marked by this repetitive cycle. Hunger, satisfaction, hunger. Pain, pain free, pain. Every night I woke up in pain and needed additional pain killers to get me through until morning.

Formerly, a high note of my day might have been a student learning from an insight achieved. Now, having lunch and dinner served to me in my room became highlights of my day. Because of my sensitivity to noise following my collision, I was unable to have my meals in the community dining area. Although my sense of isolation was profound, the simple conversation and thanks for a meal brightened my day. When friends and family stopped by occasionally to wish me well and track my progress, that too uplifted my spirits. Ironically, their visits were cut short because my level of exhaustion forced me to close my eyes and nap. My body was working so hard to repair itself I had little energy left for social interaction.

Indeed, my time away from home was lonely and disorienting.

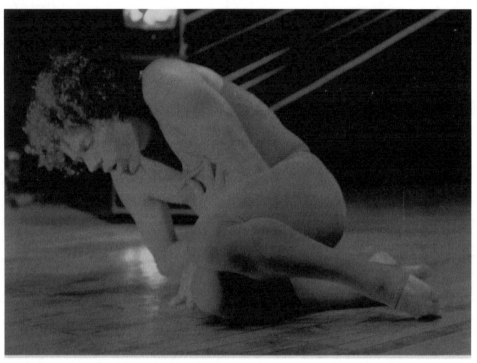

Maislen performing his "Angels Without Wings" – Artists House, NYC

Chapter Eight

WHY?

Recollection from the ICU:

"Fog. A thick soup of mist. I am not outside but there is a hum surrounding me. Have I been abducted by aliens and about to be experimented upon? I have been drugged and paralyzed. I am helpless and my fear is overwhelming."

"There are more things in heaven and earth than are dreamt of in your philosophy."
- William Shakespeare –
Hamlet

* * * *

"As you look at many people's lives, you see that their suffering is in a way gratifying, for they are comfortable in it. They make their lives a living hell, but a familiar one."
- Ram Das –
Journey of Awakening

Daily, without end, questions raced through my mind. Why did this event, accident, collision happen to me? What did I do to deserve this? Why was I singled out when there are so many evil-doers all around me who were not? There does not seem to be any justice in this event occurring. Yet, I know there is not any right or wrong. What happened simply happened!

As in Roman Polanski's movie, "Repulsion" there existed for me the feeling of a long corridor with hands appearing out of the walls viciously grabbing at me. Compounding this desperation was that the door to escape at the end of the corridor was growing more and more distant as I approached it.

The idea of thinking I was singled out could not have been further from the truth. And to allow my thoughts to question why this didn't happen to "bad" people was also deflecting me from being clear about myself. There is a fine line separating self pity from actual sadness because of loss. All the "why me" questions dancing along this line teased me into falling into a woe is me attitude. By attempting to take the higher ground, for example, and acknowledging my strength to face this disaster and overcome it, I was incrementally able to transmute the sad "why me" into the hopeful "why not me."

I wish I could go back in time, but that is impossible. Whatever has been created cannot be reversed into a time before the event. Sadly, I also discovered that there are many people worse off than I am and whose terror, loneliness, ongoing suffering and lack of comprehension makes their situation virtually unendurable.

This realization about others being worse off did not arise immediately after my traumatic event. How could it when pain and confusion lorded over me? But as the recognition of the normalcy of everyday life in people around me became more apparent, the truth of the suffering of others, for example, burns, dismemberment, blindness, paralysis, etc. produced a more constructive perspective in my mind and heart as to the "why" of my own trauma.

For my entire life, I have heard that God has a plan for us and that if we could not handle a catastrophe that befalls us, God would not have brought it to us. What does this mean? How am I supposed to reconcile my suffering with a benevolent God? How has my own free will played a part in this? And why would I have brought this upheaval into my life? How has this suffering given me greater insight into God's way? How has my estrangement from everything I thought I knew enabled me to be a better person; a more enlightened participant in this picture called life? As I healed and worked at understanding myself, many of these questions were answered.

Whether you believe in God or not, the more important point is becoming aligned with the idea that the meaning of some events are too large to comprehend. To imagine we know what God means is the height of ego. I do not know the plan. I cannot fathom the bigger picture. I do not have the ability to know what God knows.

Given this, there was great comfort in having faith that more clarity about myself would be revealed as I passed through stages of becoming healthy and strong again. This was not about "why did God choose me" but rather how can my facing a challenge increase my awareness of self and thereby help bring greater light and illumination to the world.

This did not eliminate the confusing and conflicting emotions surging through me at random moments. Rage would rise up beginning as a stumbling inside me and then rush up to the surface like an unstoppable tsunami crashing through my defenses. This intensity would be replaced by a release into acceptance that had all the earmarks of giving up. Although I was never a pushover, the combination of fear and crying made me feel as if I was shrinking into invisibility. Being helpless ate at my core and widened the gap between normalcy and my growing feeling of despair at my condition.

The confusion was my greatest enemy because it pushed and shoved me into disbelieving that hope and recovery was possible. Since answering the "why" was impossible, confusion took a prominent place in my everyday life. So letting go of trying to find an understandable niche for "why" to exist was vital to my survival. The more practical question was what steps could I take to settle the turbulent waters of confusion and enact positive healthy actions.

In fact, had I but one question, it would not be why was I chosen to experience this devastating and life altering event? Although it did not occur to my consciousness until much later, the far more significant and revealing question was: what is it within me that requires my examination?

Resources:

To Begin Again by Rabbi Naomi Levy
When Bad Things Happen to Good People by Rabbi Harold Kushner
How to go on Living When Someone You Love Dies by Therese Rando
Tear Soup by Pat Schweibert
The Tibetan Book of Living and Dying: The Spiritual Classic &
International Bestseller by Patrick Gaffney
On Death and Dying by Elisabeth Kubler-Ross

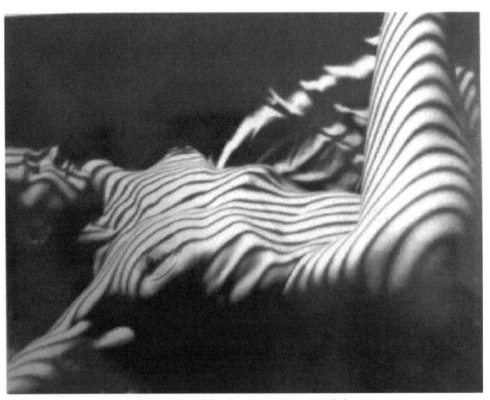

Sunshine/Shadow by Marc Maislen

PART II
GOING HOME

Chapter Nine

THE TRAUMATIZED MARRIAGE (FEBRUARY 13, 1987 - CURRENT)

Whatever the existing definition and dynamics are within a family, over time there is an ever-developing sense of the role each person is taking on or adapting to. One can be the center of attention or the laid back player in the ongoing family drama. The manner in which we interact, and what we give or receive from one another, defines the nature of our own family. If we are lucky enough to have a mom or dad who is there for us no matter what happens, we are filled with a deep sense of comfort and security in knowing we are not alone. However, at times, an unexpected event changes the climate of family life, sometimes in a moment. This can occur when a parent suddenly dies, or someone is severely injured during a war, or if a family member is struck by a disease or an accident that renders them unable to play their roles; becoming disabled or incapable of taking care of their needs. This change is almost always surprising, even shocking in its degree of separation from what represented the status quo. In my case, the collision swept away the excited anticipation my wife Mary and I felt about our new empty nest status and forced us to shelve any plans for leisure travel for an indeterminate amount of time, perhaps even forever.

The radically different picture of what family was prior to a life-altering event and what it becomes afterward cannot be adequately described. No words can even begin to touch upon the severity of stress, lack of understanding, and uncomfortable redefinition of roles that is imposed on the post-event family. No tools are given nor exercises taught in school to even remotely prepare anyone for the harshness imposed on family and the subsequent relationship shift caused by this kind of trauma.

Within the family there is the natural development of agreed upon, spoken and unspoken protocols and dynamics that emerge from the roles each member plays. But what is it that unravels and then reforms when the familiar protective barrier between individuals is shattered; when roles are no longer understood? Nothing will automatically replace the old roles we knew as family, but the pressure to establish a modicum of functionality in the face of upheaval, no matter how difficult, must be instituted.

In my case, my five grown children had already moved out of the house so I did not have the day to day experience of how my new life with disabilities would affect young, impressionable kids. What I did have was a wife, who unaccustomed to the level of stress introduced into our relationship, was trying to find a common ground between the two of us from which we could relate.

I, however, was not concerned with the dynamic changes my disability had brought about and the burdens they were creating. My attention was focused on myself; my pain and the moment to moment recovery process. I was told to work as hard as I could in getting healthy. I was not told that part of my well being was linked to Mary. No one was present to guide Mary and I through the minefield of differences now present in our relationship.

I was involved with myself. Mary was involved with herself but she was also involved with me: my pain, my anger, my questions of what was to become of me, my comfort level, and my inability to contribute physically or emotionally to the family. With all this focus on "me" and my special needs, our relationship began to suffer.

In the past when we would listen to music, the volume would be turned up very high. Now, although Mary would try to please me by playing music loudly, I would have a Post-Traumatic Stress reaction from the intensity of the sound. My emotions would become out of control and I would lash out at her or become emotionally shut down. It was not only my irrational reaction standing in isolation from the big picture that became problematic; it was also the emerging disconnection from Mary. By not acknowledging the generosity of her putting music on and by my being insensitive to her feelings by demanding the music be turned off, I was creating an ever-widening rift between us. And this is only one small example of what began happening all the time.

A caregiver takes on particular tasks and in doing so cannot always fulfill the roles previously established. The most common type of caregiver is the family caregiver: someone who takes care of a family member without pay. In dealing with tasks, for example, when Mary had to deal with my scars, my inability to get into bed or climb the stairs, my medications, my crying and my need for reassurance, the furthest activity on her mind was making love with me. By the time I was physically capable of being intimate with her, her view of me had changed. It was not so much that I was now unattractive but that in the process of her becoming my caregiver and separating herself from my unending pain, my special needs, and getting past the look of my injuries, she also had disengaged herself from sexually desiring her now unfamiliar husband.

If Mary had first met me in a rehabilitation center, her initial view of me would have been as a man with disabilities. Our growth together would have had a starting point where she understood I could not go out dancing and that I had memory problems. But we did not meet in a rehabilitation center. We met out in the world where I was a vibrant, active and mentally sharp man. I feared that this change into a person with certain limitations was also contributing to an ever-widening rift in the quality of our relationship.

Furthermore, to recognize this change required a degree of sensitivity that I, being wholly self-involved in pain, lacking sleep and adrift in confusion, was incapable of delivering. To expect my partner to remain constant in the face of my special needs was unfair. Would Mary have fallen in love with me had I started out disabled? And now that I am disabled, would my wife be able to fulfill the promise of "in sickness and in health" from our marriage vows? Many relationships cannot withstand this pressure. A deep fear began to develop as I wondered, could mine?

In another poignant example, Mary gets migraine headaches and suffers terribly from them. In our pre-collision interactions, I would do everything in my power to help her get relief from her three day ordeal. After the collision, she would not share her migraine episodes with me because she did not want to burden me. More significantly, she felt guilty to share her pain with me because "how could my pain even compare to what you are going through?" Conversely, when I had periods of lucidity I, too, would feel guilty because of my lack of contribution and the burden I was putting on her. The degree of guilt is unique to each partnership; however, this poisonous feeling was insidious and pervasive in both Mary and me. While the seeds of this guilt may be irrational, the internal destruction being rendered must be dealt with. Mary's pain was horrible and when I could no longer be a source of comfort to her, she suffered alone.

I was not betraying my wife by not being there for her. Nor was Mary purposely withholding her pain from me for some hidden agenda. We still wanted our love to grow and be as great as possible. But the repercussions of my traumatic event kept on expanding and were not limited in scope. Its impact continued to wedge itself between us. Understanding the consequences, be it guilt, sex, children, household chores or what the future holds, and taking active steps to acknowledge them, is crucial in maintaining and growing a healthy marital relationship. Sadly, for quite some time I was incapable of doing anything about any of this.

Resources:

Family Manual, A manual for families of persons with pain by Penney Cowan

Chapter Ten

CARE GIVING UP CLOSE

Three years into my recovery I unexpectedly had the opportunity of being on the opposite side of the disability fence: instead of receiving care I was called into service to give care to my ex-wife, Sandy, who was recovering from a mastectomy. When my wife and I discussed Sandy's operation and recovery we both agreed that her need was enormous and that I was the ideal candidate to help her. Mary understood how much Sandy meant to me and that my giving to her during this crisis was vital for both of us.

I might have cared for her even if I had not had a life-changing collision three years earlier but what was significant was that my new self was taking charge of the care giving. Even more interesting was the act of giving care rather than receiving it.

During the first six months after my collision, there was very little I could do for myself. I could not fully shower, wipe myself, brush my teeth, do housework, cook, or garden to name just a few. However, Mary and other friends and family members gave me the necessary care and assistance I needed so I could feel as if I was part of the household or family. God bless them!

All the little things, the minutiae of everyday living were handled by others. Normal life progressed on, albeit rougher and choppier, with the addition of speed bumps due to my collision. I never gave it much thought. More significantly, I did not take the time to examine what the almost endless number of small actions I once freely engaged in actually entailed. How much effort goes into getting a glass of water? Folding clothes from the dryer takes how long? Someone else took responsibility for these actions since I was incapable of participating in these activities. I took the execution of these tasks for granted; without recognizing and correctly thanking the caregivers surrounding me.

I moved into Sandy's spare bedroom and for two weeks I was available 24/7. Once there, I found myself having to handle the smallest of tasks because my ex-wife could not do them herself. Making a cup of tea, putting dishes in and removing them from the dishwasher, chopping vegetables for dinner, making a salad, setting the table, putting her socks on, adjusting her pillows, making sure medications were put out since the safety bottles could not be opened by her, washing her, changing the sheets and pillowcases, shopping, etc. This is a short itemization of what a caregiver needs to handle. Minor activities like turning off the light because it was time for a nap or refilling an empty glass of water became events that consumed time and energy. It is this time and energy that is at the heart of being a caregiver.

My own rehabilitation had progressed far enough that I was able to be Sandy's caregiver. I could now use both my hands, I was awakening somewhat rested from sleep, and was prescription drug free. I could walk enough to cover Sandy's house, make it easily to her doctor's appointments and stand in the kitchen to cook or do the laundry.

For the caregiver, the sense of self and personal goals becomes secondary to the patient or the one who needs to be cared for. The focus is outside of self. And in my case, after having just spent three years being the one cared for, the difference was quite a wake-up call. I can never again look at spouses, nurses, rehabilitation specialists, friends and community helpers as regular people. I will not go so far to say they are saints, but that is probably closer to the truth than any other description I would assign to them.

In recognizing what my current wife Mary did for me, it further awakened within me the connection between love, selflessness and attitude. If I could take these three elements and continually apply them in my life, I would find myself growing in remarkable ways because of the power inherent in these qualities. In acknowledging what Mary did for me I was able to deepen the relationship between us. And in becoming the care giver for Sandy I was able to experience the difficulty in sustaining selfless giving, the struggle to continually pay attention to someone else in need, and the sharpening of sensitivity in the sense that I had to develop the ability to anticipate her needs and desires so I would be prepared when something happened and not be caught off guard.

By becoming involved in care giving I understood how precious personal time is because so little of it was available for me. The moment I sat down and relaxed, another demand was voiced that needed to be addressed. I might think could that demand have waited? Or, could a few demands be bunched together and asked at a later moment? Of course that is possible. But the ailing person is not considering others; they are self absorbed, and rightfully so. The lesson for me (and for others who have been in the position of needing care) is that the caregiver deserves respect and acknowledgement as an integral contributor to the healing process even if the patient is incapable of expressing it well. All the little things I did alone and all the activities that my wife and I previously did together were now being done by her alone. The value of this selflessness needs to be understood and the one rendering this service needs to be thanked.

On a personal level, because I had dealt with being immobilized, I could help Sandy understand that her inability to raise her arm over her head would pass. I had also grown in self compassion and self acceptance because of living with tremendous pain, so I could comfort her when she felt "less than" and when she felt guilty that she needed to medicate to experience relief.

My ex-wife was deeply grateful to me for making the time to take care of her and be with her unconditionally. What I came away with was the understanding that the caregiver is contributing almost as much time and energy as the injured person in the recovery process and to not judge the capabilities of the injured person.

Resources:

The Fearless Caregiver: How to Get the Best Care for Your Loved One and Still Have a Life of Your Own (Capital Cares) by Gary Barg
God Knows Caregiving Can Pull You Apart: 12 Ways to Keep it All Together by Gretchen Thompson
Caregiving: The Spiritual Journey of Love, Loss, and Renewal by Beth Witrogen McLeod

Chapter Eleven

COMPANIONSHIP

The overwhelming sense of hopelessness, experienced alone, can quickly erode any gains. There are twenty four hours in a day and only so many of these hours can be spent participating in active recovery. What is the quality of life during the down times? What is the mind going through when not focused on a recovery exercise? What thoughts dominate and color the way in which we look at ourselves and the world?

Without a partner willing to walk through the minefield of victories and defeats alongside you, the grind of daily chores, day-to-day activities, and open-ended unfilled time, the burden of life can weigh so heavily that any sense of fluidity can become impossible. The simple act of talking to my wife, especially during stretches of confusion and pain became an oasis of hope that never wavered. The haven of comfort and understanding that my wife supplied was the touchstone that enabled me to safely return to a positive state on a daily basis.

When Mary would gently hold my damaged right hand and knead my fingers, I felt a sense that my heart was being touched. It was as if she was "milking" my hand, my fingers like teats, so that I could feel my core, my basic life energy moving down through my hand and co-mingling with her energy.

Every couple's relationship is unique in its own way. For Mary and I, theatre, performing, and the search for a core truth were our fundamental pillars. We related to each other as warriors and respected each others' paths to understanding. We never treated each other as "I do this better than you" but rather "we bring different strengths to each other and the task at hand." The wealth of unspoken acceptance and respect had a profound weight, giving value to our ability to share. We understood that although we suffer alone, the gift of comforting each other was far more valuable than mentally trying to out think the problem.

I was fortunate to not be abandoned by my wife after my collision. However, many severely injured people are left to weather the storm alone. To draw friends or other family members into the circle of healing is critical to continued mental health. Since so much time is spent in solitary recovery, the value of sharing the impediments, challenges and changes being dealt with are invaluable additions to the healing process.

When my friend Mike came to my house for SuperBowl 2007, his presence was invigorating. We were able to share a common activity without any focus on my bodily damages. I was treated like just another friend, a regular person cheering for my team, eating mini hot dog smokies and guzzling beer. More importantly, I was not watching the game alone.

A different element in companionship is a pet. My dog, Willow, exhibited the unconditional love that only a dog can. Not only was she exuberant when she visited me during my month long stay in the recovery home but her devotion once I returned home was beautiful.

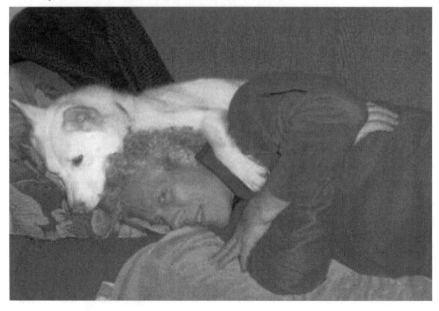

When you pet a dog there is actually more happening than just the dog feeling your hand on its fur. Science has shown that a subtle energy is given back to you from the dog when you pet them[3]. During recovery this exchange of energy gently soothes the damaged body. This certainly was true for me.

My dog would sit for many hours right next to me on the couch as my body was propped up by various pillows. The number of hours I spent on that couch over the course of the first two years was made infinitely more meaningful (and bearable) because of her presence. I now recognize the difference in her participation because since I have recovered enough to be mobile again, she only spends a limited amount of time lying next to me when I sit on the couch.

I think that as a wolf dog, Willow's pack instincts were on high alert. My general physical absence and overall mental distance kicked Willow's mothering instincts into gear and gave her a reason to be, a role-playing member of the tribe. What was so interesting was that no human would consider "just laying there" for hours and days on end. But she did. And where taking a drug relaxed my body, Willow's warmth and actual body to body contact gave me a comfort no medication could duplicate.

While so much recovery time is experienced alone, the shared time, emotional support, and unconditional love given by a partner and/or animal is an invaluable asset in bridging the gap between isolation, feeling cut off from people, and connecting in order to feel part of humanity. Since the goal after a life-threatening event is to integrate as fully as possible back into the world, this contribution to recovery cannot be understated.

3 Neurophysiiological correlates of affiliative behaviour between humans and dogs. Odendaal JS, Meintjes RA. Vet J. 2003 May; 165(3):296-301

Chapter Twelve

EXPECTATION

Finally, the expectations I set up for myself were a double-edged sword. Having the hopefulness and expectation of improvement is a positive use of attitude. However, when an expectation is shattered, the internal reaction can be devastating. The truth of what IS must be consciously dealt with. Additionally, part of the stability of family rests on the expectation that the individual members will act within a range of expectation.

One month prior to my collision my daughter, Marissa, began her college career at NYU Tisch School of Dance. For years I would assist her in homework assignments and critique her dance performances. After watching her dance classes I gave her feedback and helped demonstrate challenging dance combinations. Marissa came to rely on me for insights into her progress. The distress and emptiness she felt, being abandoned in a way by my unavailability, caused her profound loneliness and produced a fundamental change in our relationship.

Similarly, my son, Adam, living in Seattle at the time, after visiting me in the ICU was so upset he could not return to the hospital. Where prior to my collision we would spend many hours playing cards and discussing poker strategy, now I was unable to concentrate effectively or use our card playing as a relationship building activity. Adam's expectation of his father as a source of strength, confidence and insight dissolved into a picture of a man who was incapable of taking care of himself.

Finally, Mary's emotional life was intertwined with mine in a stable, intimate fashion. Prior to my collision we would share thoughts, feelings, future possibilities, and the creative world of theatre and dance in which both of us were active participants. After the collision, Mary was reluctant to voice emotions she was experiencing since I was too self involved to listen or too disconnected to effectively present alternative possibilities. Having to isolate her feelings without expressing them was diametrically opposed to the way in which she had led her life. Additionally, ongoing conversations about art, creativity and theatre/dance productions came to a screeching halt. Any expectation Mary had for me to openly receive her ideas and thoughts were finished. What changes in her behavior, intellectual exchanges or intimacy did she have to go through? What words could she speak without fearing an anxiety reaction from me? How would she fill in the communication gaps between us? And what would she do to stabilize the static and uncertainty of her husband no longer being a solid provider?

The sheer number of past patterns and expectations my wife and I once seamlessly acted upon now appeared as hurdles on our path. The answer rested on how effectively my wife could streamline and simplify daily activities. Scheduling revolved around my doctors' and hospital appointments. Results were weighed not in the timeliness of getting chores completed but in the fact that the chores could be accomplished at all.

While many of these expectations found new ways to be resolved, and as I recovered my abilities to some degree, I planned on visiting my mother and two of my children in New York. I projected that I would be able to function well enough to handle the travel as well as getting around the city, not as a typical fast paced New Yorker as I had always been, but rather as a person recovering from a near-fatal collision who would move at a slower pace giving myself extra time to get from place to place.

As the time drew closer for my departure I realized that making such a strenuous trip would not be possible. Was my family going to be disappointed that I could not make the trip? What did I feel about not being able to go? What was I going to do and how was I going to handle this?

Having to cancel the much anticipated trip, I could have easily slipped back into depression with its commensurate lessening of self worth. Instead, I chose to honestly look at myself and evaluate what I saw. This was a difficult and painful moment of truth for me which required some real soul-searching. I needed to admit that I was not capable of such a physically taxing adventure and more importantly I needed to forgive myself for both not being able to make the trip and for disappointing others.

Time and again, I was discovering that the need to drop an expectation and replace it with a more realistic scenario is a necessary ingredient in making a healthy recovery. While I wanted to be more active and healthy, this desire could not always be fulfilled in my predetermined time frame. Overcoming this idea of "how much time" things now took was a freeing experience. To be willing to adjust and be happy with the modified behavior or activity is crucial in making the incremental changes necessary for a long lasting, permanent recovery.

Resources:

Coping With Family Expectations by Margaret Hill

Chapter Thirteen

BRAIN ON HOLD

Dreamlike recollection from the ER:

"There is a churning sea beneath me; angry foam screaming as it tries to swallow me. I am desperately clinging to the slippery rungs of a ladder. A child clutches my ankle. The rung above me is safety but I must allow the ever weakening grasp of the child to be swallowed up into the turbulent sea if I am to survive."

* * * * *

"I have buried disappointments in the cemeteries of yesterday. Today I will plow the garden of life with my new creative efforts. Therein I will sow seeds of wisdom, health, prosperity and happiness. I will water them with self-confidence and faith, and will wait for the Divine to give me the rightful harvest."
- Paramahansa Yogananda –

The effects of my brain injury were instantaneously apparent. The most immediate being my inability to remember the crash.

During the first six months after my collision I was constantly reminded of my brain damage. There were multiple indicators of brain trauma from acute to subtle. My first recognition of a problem was the left side of my face not moving the way the right side moved. I can only imagine and wonder in disbelief why people injecting Botox would do such a thing. My muscles did not respond nearly as well on the left side of my face. The worst facet of this powerlessness was my left lower lip sagging, unable to form words correctly. It felt as if I had a flubber lip. This lip problem was combined with my inability to speak double "L"s. Speaking any word ending in "lly" came out as a growly 'lrrr' sound, causing me to stop and force my tongue and lip to form a double "L".

This condition persisted for well over a year, getting incrementally better.

What was shocking and very disturbing was having the loss of vocabulary. In the middle of a conversation I would have to repeatedly stop to ask the speaker what a word meant. Simple words like 'travel' or 'tunnel' or 'rose' or 'green' to name a few, were unrecognizable by me. I was constantly asking my wife and others to define many common words. As an avid crossword puzzle solver my level of frustration was enormous. But right from the onset of recovery my neurologist recommended reading as much as possible and to keep trying to do crosswords. The current understanding of brain-neuroscience indicates the brain will re-pattern itself and find new neural pathways when stimulations are repeatedly attempted.[4] What began as frustrating and anger producing crossword puzzle attempts became an exciting challenge. I felt both as a child and as a stroke victim: learning language from ground zero. Additionally, whenever I tried to speak quickly or when I was getting more emotionally engaged, I would stutter. This verbal dysfunction persisted for about four years, slowly getting less troublesome over time.

The most disturbing brain damage was the wiping out of random long-term memories. For me it was understandable that I had no recollection of my collision but is was not acceptable that I had lost all memory of my first trip to Paris or what happened to the theatre set pieces from my first show. Many interactions and memories of people and friends were gone as if they had never existed. This condition continued during the first year and lingers to a lesser extent now resulting in a sad and empty feeling of loss. There is a hole where a memory once existed.

Secondary to the full blown memory loss was a marked decrease in short-term memory. If my wife asked me to get cheese from the refrigerator I would open the fridge door and not have a clue as to what I was looking for. Or during rehab sessions I simply could not remember how many sets I had done. Markedly problematic at the onset of recovery, I have since adopted a manageable device of writing down simple tasks, instructions and thoughts. This way I can return to them and reference them later, however, this problem still persists.

Many friends say that both of the above conditions are simply part of the aging process. I know this to be untrue. There is a difference between trying to remember something knowing it exists somewhere (normal people) versus searching for the memory or reference point and finding a void (brain damage). Knowing certain events happened but all that remains is a hole and a blank where that memory should have been, is not the same as forgetting. This is so difficult to describe but still persists as a "nothingness" and remains uncomfortable and disconcerting.

The last obvious brain trauma was my new inability to hold multiple thoughts at the same time as well as the resulting feeling engendered by this occurrence. The immediate post-collision reaction was when noise or sound became too loud I would have an anxiety attack. The other post-collision aspect was when conversation became varied with multiple inputs by a group of friends and I would become confused and agitated. I became incapable of actually hearing what was being spoken and I became "glazed over" by dissociating from the activity and the vibration of too much stimulation. It felt as if my brain compartments were no longer present, had changed dimension or were being blocked. I could no longer multitask or run an emotional high to the fullest degree without becoming shut down. I had always identified myself as someone who could carry multiple ideas and conversations simultaneously; like a chess master playing ten games blindfolded at once. This incapacity made me feel confused and evoked feelings of stupidity and inadequacy.

Nonetheless, I knew that no matter how frustrating my lack of brain response and sketchy memory recognition was manifesting, I would not give up. I worked on reprogramming my brain and remaining open to learning new ways to experience life. It took well over two years before I successfully completed a crossword puzzle. As for other aspects, reframing memories and being in the "now" for loud and active experiences remains an on-going challenge.

Chapter Fourteen

FEAR AND THE WALL

My recollection on Flashbacks:

"It's great getting out to the movies. I'm feeling very comfortable watching 'The Lookout.' Suddenly the lead character is in a devastating crash with a truck. My hands are vice-gripping the arms of the seat. My back is pinned against the chair. My mouth is frozen, gaping open. Oh, this is not comfortable being triggered this way."

* * * *

"The more we try to struggle, the more we will discover that walls really are solid. The more energy we put into struggle, by that much will we strengthen the walls, because the walls need our attention to solidify them."

\- Chogyam Trungpa –
Cutting Through Spiritual Materialism

In my pre-catastrophe life I functioned with some semblance of confidence and without a separation between myself and the world. The interplay of events and actions flowed seamlessly. But whether I adhered to or disregarded the outside world's judgment about how sick or well I was, the after effect of my life-changing event was that I became more fearful of the outside world. At times, I even perceived an imaginary barrier or wall, an impediment between myself and the world around me.

Fear is invisible, unseen or hidden and yet it represents an emotion that can debilitate even the strongest amongst us. If I intellectually approach fear as the opposite of love, the simplistic resolution to the onset of fear is to love more fully. In fact, this is a solution to the problem. However, the application of love required far more than lip service or an intellectual understanding.

I had been altered by a catastrophic event and this alteration affected the way I saw myself. I was weaker physically and no longer felt I could protect myself or my family. To compound the problem, this changed view also allowed fear to take root. For me, the world itself and its people became more threatening. To protect myself from my escalating fear of the world, I insulated myself by erecting a wall of protection to create a buffer zone. A simple deception was telling myself that I really did not want to go out. That kept me in the house. Or saying it would be too crowded at a gathering. That choice assured I would be house bound. Unfortunately, rather than helping me, this strategy created a secondary problem. I now had a wall in addition to fear.

How was I to handle this? I recognized that first I had to examine my fear.

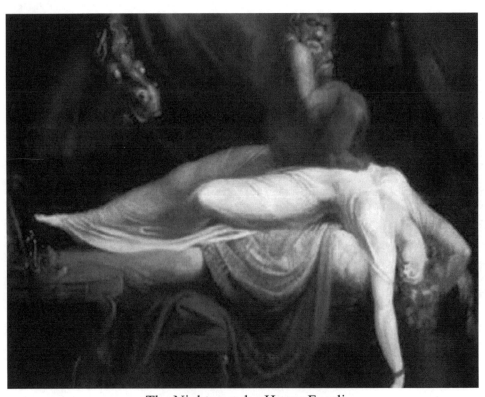

The Nightmare by Henry Fuseli

Chapter Fifteen

SINKING

My recollection on 9/11:

"It is the anniversary of the attack on 9/11. All I can feel is being trapped in my car. I feel such a pressure on my chest that it is difficult to breathe. I am scared of being unable to move because of the weight. I can't get past the feeling of being trapped and being powerless to do anything about it. What did the victims go through? What suffering did they experience? Someone alive and trapped...."

* * * *

"No healing can take place until we decide to think actively about the dark side. Each of us has a dark side."
                                                              - Robert Bly –

When a life altering event takes place, replete with trauma and pain, and with a prognosis of permanent damage, the brain does not quietly assemble these pieces together. The brain does not serenely slide into acceptance. The mind does not adopt the severity of these issues as if nothing had happened. If anything, the brain refuses to accept the new reality and tries to block out portions of the truth. One segment of the brain's masking of reality is the thought of turning it all off: suicide.

If someone told me I would be considering suicide, I probably would have laughed them out of the room. Certainly some people are religiously opposed to suicide while others feel a moral obligation to preserve life at all costs. My experience has nothing to do with God, religion, morality or judgment. My thoughts of suicide originated from the depth of my pain, despair, and hopelessness.

Overcoming suicidal thoughts required gaining strength in the face of overwhelming challenges and honestly examining myself as I confronted the barriers of impossibility. These realizations lit the fire of commitment for me to want to be alive.

My darkness was like a nightmare. It made me feel as if I was in a perfectly designed sleek metal cage; each strut and crosspiece joined in simplicity and balance. Like a bad dream, I am walking inside this trap, discovering that it is a giant hamster wheel, its movement determined by my speed. Running, racing to escape, I can only remain in place, energy being siphoned off like the ground wire of conductivity. My reward, the morsels of food awaiting my consumption, is reached when I balance the wheel and stretch my arm to its furthest extreme without creating any disturbing motion. Clearly I am not in control because this dark world is about settling in the cage while I remain committed to gaining sustenance from the nurturing provisions. Nonetheless, this bleakness will never allow me to forget that I am trapped in the cage.

It is easy to say that we are on Earth for a purpose; that our lives mean something. But when everything I knew was forever altered and the overarching pain of being alive was relentless, the idea of my purpose on Earth became bleak. The old picture of life flowing smoothly no longer had relevance, so my ability to focus on purpose lost its meaning. When existence loses relevance, suicide is not an unreasonable thought.

My thoughts of suicide never grabbed me like a vicious fighter would, with one strong hand gripping my throat. Rather, these thick thoughts produced fissures where my shattered dreams seeped through to reveal all the feelings of hopelessness and of never again being happy or whole. These thoughts prevented the slightest pinprick of hopeful light to breathe through.

There is an unsettling image of gasps of air burning my lungs in a frantic and fearful arrhythmic desperation. What is giving up and giving in to suicide? What part of self is beheaded when the great ax falls? The pervasive nature of bleakness can be like a magnet, that growing in power attracts and amasses more futility. Is that suicide?

After my car crash, my insecurities mounted. This growing despair, this increasing weight of despondency upon my chest, was the daily judgment of discovering my feet then ankles then knees were being imperceptibly sucked into quicksand. Is this image of being swallowed up, seen out of the corner of my eye in the shadows, the hidden specter of suicide?

Thoughts of suicide grew in me with suffocating regularity. Like an incurable rash, every inch of skin that might have remained smooth was ultimately covered, obscuring any windows into life, leaving only darkness. The absolute zero of hope is suicide and therein rested my escape from this hell. The final prognosis of suicide is relief, where the nothing is.

Depression goes hand in hand with thoughts of suicide. When I was feeling positive and hopeful, I was not depressed and therefore not building up suicidal thoughts. In my former life I had good days and bad days. But in my new reality, it was much easier to have a series of bad days or bad weeks in a row. Once I had a bad day, it was that much more difficult to get a foothold and climb out of it because my pool of inner resources was so depleted. Once this negative spiral begins, attempting to reverse this trend is very problematic. The layers of buried memories, the rust of old patterns, the flashes of desires unfulfilled, all impeded my own worthiness to love myself.

So when I examined the pool of resources available to me, it became apparent that it was vital to expand my vision to include more than my immediate, self-evident limited abilities. What I mean by this is that I had to be open to a more unlimited potential, where a broader range of human possibilities could become a usable resource. For some this possibility is God. For me this meant tapping into the Source. This shift in thinking kick started a more hopeful attitude and made it possible for me to reverse the suicidal trend I had fallen into.

I recognized I could not make this shift alone so I sought out a psychotherapist to help facilitate this transition. I went for weekly and sometimes twice weekly sessions. It is quite miraculous what benefits can be accomplished by participating in regular sessions with a trained mental health professional. I know it was for me. In addition, depression and suicide are often treated with medication. I chose to integrate Wellbutrin into my healing plan until it was no longer necessary.

It is natural to have emotional and mental reactions to trauma. Just as I sought help in repairing my physical body, seeing a psychotherapist helped realign my mental body. What I found helpful was learning how to address the problems I was experiencing more objectively. When I was able to see the problems clearly I began to stabilize and improve myself.

A meaningful example of how I was being helped was when I was rambling on about how angry and frustrated I was about not being able to move in the way I was accustomed to. Instead of allowing me to generally complain, my therapist asked what I missed the most. As I began to talk about bicycling I could not control my tears. Further inquiry into the root of my sadness was that my "loss" was less about my inability to pedal but the feeling that I was no longer free. I felt inadequate and reliant on others to get me through the world. When she enabled me to see and feel that others helped me manage the quagmire of the world by giving their love, not through obligation, I was able to embrace the feeling of "sharing freedom" instead of having to do it all myself. What a powerful breakthrough! By reshaping my ideas of isolation from an attitude of loneliness into a belief of sharing I could open up my heart. For example, where my old view of bicycling was one person to a bike, this new picture revealed a tandem, where two people ride on a bike. I saw, and subsequently experienced my wife and I enjoying this together. This was a breakthrough for me.

Another problem I faced was acute anxiety. We have all experienced moments of confusion but when I was first getting acclimated to my new self these moments of confusion could last for many minutes and were out of my control. This was especially apparent when I was not in the comfort zone of my own home but out in the world. For me, the world sometimes appeared to be moving at a speed that defied comprehension. My new self was moving more slowly than before because it was trying to adjust to my new way of being. But the world was not slowing down for me. I, who had always been a quick thinker, found myself mentally registering a world that was moving too fast for me to understand. Also, since I was not fluidly interacting with the world, the combination of the two created an inner experience of high anxiety. Again, I was grateful I had a therapist to assist me in understanding what was happening so I could handle the stress and ultimately progress through it.

However, even though I was seeing a mental health professional, I still had thoughts of suicide. When I looked at the burden I was imposing on my wife, I thought one way to free her from this weight was to take my own life. But I felt that this way out, similar to other rationales leading to this conclusion, was still a cowardly act. My spouse may have had reasons to walk out on me, but I had no right to walk out on myself.

The turning point came when a fellow performer called me to ask if I was well enough to begin staging my children's story. Although I was not ready to tackle a theatre project, I realized I certainly was not prepared to leave one of my "writing babies" in the lurch. I owed it to myself and to my wife to see this through. The skewed thinking process that by taking my own life it freed others now made no sense.

When I focused on the important goals in my life and the tasks I could perform, I gained new and vital reasons for living. When I began to believe I could find new interests, I discovered a wealth of avenues opening up for me to pursue. This was crucial for me in rekindling my desire to live.

There was an ever-expanding sliver of light that illuminated hopelessness into a powerful drive of hope. While I could not see hope as a single continuous presence, staying aligned with the process of finding hope in even small things, like starting to pronounce the letter "L" or adding five pounds to a leg curl, highlighted the idea that suicide was a lack of trust in myself. The light was focused on me trusting greater things were going to come.

Slowly, and then with increasing clarity, I began to realize that this period of recovery was a time to gain strength in the face of adversity, not a time to give up. I realized that this was a time to look clearly at myself without backing down from the severity of the hurdles I needed to overcome.

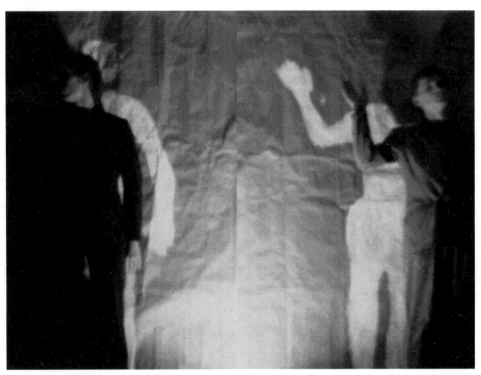

Marc Maislen/Michael Simon – AvantGardeArama PS 122, NYC

PART III
DOING THE WORK

Chapter Sixteen

COMMITTING TO RECOVERY

My recollection on Physical Therapy:

"This can't be happening. This simple movement, this "clam shell," of opening my hip by raising my knee is agonizing. Not just one time but over and over again. I am struggling to cope with my lack of motion and the pain. This is such an easy movement and I can't do it."

* * * *

"The moment one definitely commits oneself, then Providence moves, too. All sorts of things occur to help one that would never otherwise have occurred...Boldness has genius, power, and magic in it. Begin it now."

- Johann Wolfgang von Goethe -

When I was a teenager I was care free about life and cavalier about my abilities. If I could get away with minimal studying for an exam, that was the time I put in. If I convinced myself that hitting tennis forehands using one basket of balls was quite enough for the day, I walked away satisfied with my effort. In retrospect the only person I was deceiving was myself.

Now at this critical juncture in my life if I try to take shortcuts and refuse to make a commitment to recovery, there is no magic wand that will help me. If I waltz into physical therapy with the expectation that the therapist is going to manipulate me into health, I am in store for a rude awakening. Without decisively committing to exercise during the "off hours" I know I will never recover. And exercise in the off hours does not necessarily mean hundreds of push-ups or sit-ups. It could mean opening and closing my hand and stretching my fingers four to five times a day; or squeezing my butt cheeks together whenever I am watching TV. It may be boring and unglamorous but these repetitions are the crucial ingredients in making a dynamic change in muscle strength and flexibility. Being honest with myself was not easy but I did not have the luxury of kidding around. By committing to these repetitions I knew I could ultimately add more difficulty and variety to my recovery program.

My dream/reality comes even closer as I see the barbells and weights in the rehab center. I see the dynabands, balls, pulleys, bikes, treadmills, and pieces of equipment. I breathe in my amazement of where I am. I breathe out my fear of using this equipment. I am not confined in the rehab space. I slowly approach the barbell and touch it. I am struck by how cool it is against my skin. I gently push against it and I feel the resistance of its weight. I breathe in my readiness. I lift the weight and my body engages. I feel the electricity in my body. I breathe in and smile. There is nothing else but me, working, working hard. My muscles are responding. I am alive. I breathe in hope and excitement. I am living my participation in my own destiny. This is a good thing. I breathe in and smile.

Let's not fool ourselves. The commitment is work. For me the commitment is not giving up when the exercises become painful. The commitment is doing the work when I am not motivated to get up and go to the gym, or even when I do not want to stretch my body. The commitment is being kind and respectful to myself by giving myself the permission to work hard and then allowing myself the time to recover as fully as possible. The commitment is having the belief that my recovery program is worth the struggle. The commitment even produces the feeling of being uplifted because it honors what I am doing as a valid activity.

I know how grueling this work is. I also realize not everyone can work so hard. I never woke in the morning looking forward to being a beast in rehab because I knew that this challenge is so difficult it is understandable to not push so intensely. Having gone through hundreds of hours of training to become a dancer I could relate to what effort it took to repeatedly pound my body. I'm sure construction workers can understand this but office workers might not understand or get behind the validity of such an effort. The commitment is starting at whatever level you're at and then affirming "I really will try 100%." Using my physical therapist to the fullest extent and taking extra sessions in the rehab gym made a huge difference.

Commitment starts with me but very often it entails allowing another person, generally a health care professional to be close to me, especially when they need to touch my body. By having them in such close proximity to me, my willingness to be physically manipulated is tested. Can I trust this person to move various parts of my body when those movements are painful? There is a deep sense of vulnerability in allowing that professional person in. Talk about intimacy! My aura of self protectiveness had to be slightly unguarded, and the feeling that they are so close to me that their breath and intention is wafting into my nose is often difficult to accept.

Yet, the feeling of allowing someone in goes far past a simple welcoming cue. In real life I make a tacit agreement to be friendly that short circuits protectiveness; but I do not open up so wide that I am at risk. The positive aspect of opening up is that this gateway not only allows the new to enter myself but enables the weary mustiness of my old and unhelpful thoughts to escape. So the questions become: When my armor is bombarded by injury and destruction, what will my choice be? Will I embrace the outstretched hand of a friend and know it is the lifeline of recovery? Will I recognize these professionals and friends as they step up to the plate? And will I reveal my own vulnerability by opening up and asking for help?

It is so easy to simply say "yes" to these questions. But my life did not prepare me for blanket acceptance. My life did not foster trust and belief in the kindness of others. I had to truly look at myself, albeit in my damaged state, and find my willingness to change.

When I was healthy I pushed my physical limits practicing the mantra, "no pain, no gain." When I became a personal trainer I learned this regimen invites hurting oneself when the body is trying to tell you to stop the activity. Nonetheless, my rehabilitation process needed to embrace that concept. However, it was equally important for me to recognize when the pain I experienced was actually hurting me. Plus, it was difficult telling the person I was trusting to help me that the exercises were too much. At times I pushed too hard and I came away with injuries and an inability to continue my rehab program until the injuries healed. One time this happened during unsupervised rehab when I lifted too much weight doing bicep curls and strained my muscles. Although I could not return to rehab for several days, I knew that "no pain, no gain" was an accurate assessment of what was required of me in order to produce the results I desired.

After years of dancing, extending fully and leaping through space, it shocked me that when I exercised any injured part of my body, it would not want to move very far. My skills and joy of motion went out the window. Now I was going to have to force the movement in order to increase the range of motion. Being injured, when I push past my comfortable range, the part of my body I am exercising is going to hurt. Knowing this fact does not make it easier but I understand this pain is acceptable and necessary. If I refuse to make the commitment to work through this pain, I will not make any gain in my range of motion. I am focused on the purpose of my rehabilitation: to come as close as possible to my previous ability or as close as possible to what would be considered normal.

As there is less dream and more reality I become excited in the gym. I breathe. I am lifting light weights or gently stretching my muscles. I breathe in and feel a renewed connection with my body. I am so far from the dark and lonely place and I feel good. I still can't move very much but it feels all right. The therapist has a big smile. All is well. I breathe in confidence. Then the therapist adds more weight and my work becomes more difficult. Suddenly I don't feel so well. My heart starts racing and my vision begins narrowing. I am not feeling comfortable. The pain is kicking in. I am confused. My therapist is saying "you can do it." I breathe in with anger. I breathe in the acceptance of the pain. I am determined. I will succeed. I will do these exercises. I breathe in energy and I exhale a feeling of completion. I am on the correct road.

Like most activities in life there is no single way that works for everyone. I needed to keep my progress in perspective because damage is relative to each individual. Someone having a heart attack and going through rehab is significantly different than me having hip reconstruction surgery. The program of rehabilitative work is relative to the trauma and resultant damage. Attempting to walk after a heart attack is quite different from me walking after hip surgery. My attempt at walking after hip surgery entailed localized pain (in the hip joint) and the surrounding muscles that are taking the brunt of force when walking. When I worked next to someone after their heart attack the overarching weakness in their body prevented them from having a steady, strong walk.

My pain/gain after hip reconstruction surgery was indeed fighting through the pain in order to increase strength within the joint to allow an easier, pain free walk. The pain/gain after a heart attack might be more general (the entire body hurts) until strength and a stronger blood flow is built up which produces more endurance. In both cases, even though the pain is different and localized (hip) versus non-local (body), one must progress through the pain by increasing strength.

Even though my injuries are causing the pain, what I have come to understand is increased strength will help alleviate the pain. This improved strength is what freed me from pain; naturally coupling with the previous idea that commitment will help free me from pain. Nonetheless, the act of being committed while taking responsibility for my rehabilitation was still not enough. The creeping feeling of being "less than" or fundamentally "weak" as a result of having been injured also had to be battled. I had to remember that even though I needed to build my strength, this current weakness was not the cause of my pain. So I spoke to myself with a new mantra: I am injured, not weak. Therefore, the building of strength is two-fold: it is positive reinforcement (I can see my muscles getting stronger) and it also assists me in overcoming the trauma I have experienced (stronger equals less pain).

I find it ironic that having experienced agonizing pain during the traumatic event I now must experience another threshold of pain in order to return to normal. Yet, if I am unwilling to pass through the pain barrier and maintain a strong "work ethic," I will be unable to make my new self as healthy as possible.

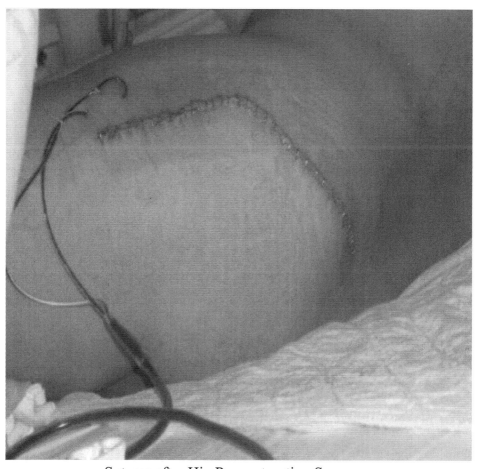

Sutures after Hip Reconstruction Surgery

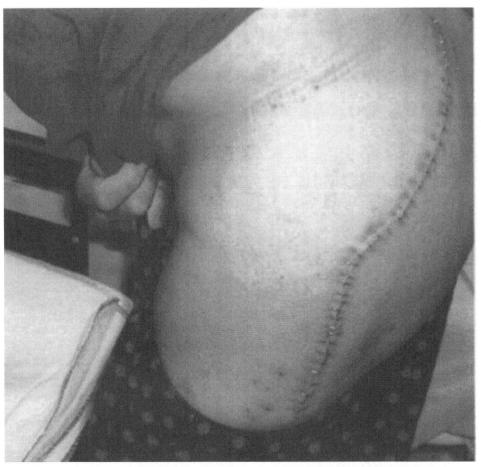

What a Permanent Scar after Hip Surgery will look like

Chapter Seventeen

MOTIVATION

My recollection on taking a Shower:

"After discharge from the hospital and admission to a rehab facility I have yet to shower. I can't walk or use my arm and hand so doing this by myself is out of the question. Etta offers her services to me and I gratefully accept. Wheeled into the shower, helped into a shower chair and sitting naked, I am embarrassed. But once this great nurse begins to set the water temperature and wash me I finally have a feeling that is pleasurable. What a simple joy to feel clean and showered. The water is magnificent."

* * * *

"Very seldom will a person give up on himself. He continues to have hope because he knows he has the potential for change. He tries again – not just to exist but to bring about those changes in himself that will make his life worth living."
- Hugh Prather –
Notes on Love and Courage

If I was asked to summarize myself prior to my collision I would have said I was a mature, energetic, intelligent and funny person. So what was I left with after the facade of my old self image was stripped away after my catastrophic event? Simply, I was left with my naked self. Unfortunately, there is no guarantee that once we are face to face with our self that we will be happy with whom we see. This was the case with me. The only thread I could cling to was the possibility that this new emerging self would be stronger and wiser because of all I had gone through.

It was actually exciting to find that becoming aware of the unpleasant parts of myself and seizing the opportunity to redefine them, was a built-in motivational tool. In the face of all my damage, there was no expectation for me to be my old self. Now, instead of being a bit of a lone wolf, I was choosing to welcome people in and listen attentively. This resulted in people opening up and trusting me more. In the midst of my recovery I was actually gaining friends!

It seemed that by not worrying about my appearance, after all I was a mess with stitches and scars, I was also not concerned with what others thought about me. Once freed from these worries I found my interest was piqued in others. Before my collision I felt I needed to tell my story. Since my story was plain to see and I was in the moment, I was now available to fill my cup with the stories and emotions of others, many of whom in far worse shape than me. By listening and absorbing what was said, I found myself inspired by their challenges. This motivated my growth.

When examining the stripped down version of myself, I also uncovered qualities in myself that I respected. I was proud of my bulldog tenacity. This quality could be useful in motivating me through painful rehab sessions or in doggedly holding onto the desire to be whole again. In examining the depression and hopelessness that gnawed at me, my tenacity could overcome these feelings and motivate my new self into being positive, resilient and healthy. And this tenacity is exactly what I used.

My dream/reality takes on a different shape as I breathe in and look at myself. Who is staring back at me? I wonder whether I like the person in the mirror. I breathe in my whole self. I breathe out any old useless parts of myself. I recognize that I am strong in my own way. I smile knowing others are willing to see the new me. I smile knowing I am surprising myself. I breathe in my possibilities. This strength is driving me on. I am motivated by me. I breathe in and look at myself. I know I am motivated to do whatever it takes.

I recollect many years before when I went on a five day Vipassana Meditation Retreat in western Massachusetts. I took a vow of silence and the only activity I engaged in was sitting, with the focus on bringing awareness to my breath. I discovered where the breath comes from, how it enters the lungs and fills the body, and how all tension can be released on the exhale. This was an invaluable tool I used daily during each stage of my recovery. The simplicity of breathing with awareness helped both in diminishing my pain and in releasing tension from my body. I was so grateful that this process spurred on an ever deepening level of motivation to persevere.

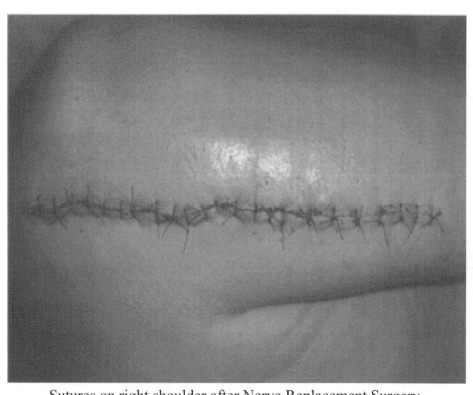

Sutures on right shoulder after Nerve Replacement Surgery

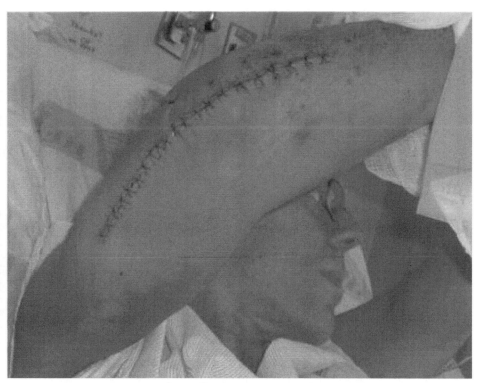

Sutures after Elbow Reconstruction Surgery

Chapter Eighteen

COURAGE

My recollection on Courage:

"I was confined to a wheelchair. Now I was allowed to put 1/8 of my weight on my leg. I was terrified to put too much weight on it and yet thrilled that I was standing and moving my damaged leg. I wanted to cross the room. I needed to get to the opposite wall. I knew I would eventually walk there unassisted."

* * * *

"Courage is the price that Life exacts for granting peace."
        - Amelia Earhart –

* * * *

"Life shrinks or expands according to one's courage."
        - Anais Nin –

The textbook definition of courage is the quality of spirit that enables you to face danger or pain without showing fear; the mettle, spirit and tenacity of mental strength to resist hardship.

These descriptive words give meaning to this intangible quality of courage. While a soldier's valor in the fierceness of battle is a brazen act of courage, the battle I face every day on the minefield of recovery is no less courageous.

This kind of courage was never more evident the first time I attempted to get into bed by myself after my collision. I understood that unless I was able to overcome the pain, I would be unable to maneuver through this seemingly simple act. Similarly, I had to sit on each riser in order to get up the steps in my house. I could not walk more than one block. I could not reach the top shelf or wash my hair and my hand could neither grasp nor hold even a lightweight object.

The pain of moving my body required me to have the courage to face the pain and to relentlessly persevere in not giving up. It was far easier to remain pain free – by not moving. I knew I didn't want to be the frightened deer frozen in place awaiting the onrushing car. There was no way I would be willing to spend the rest of my life frozen in place. So like a clever trickster I had to coax the damaged, non-moving parts into a reasonable range of motion. The courage to face the pain, embrace it, battle it, and subdue it is no less courageous than a soldier fighting in a war zone.

Is it possible to relate to "The Little Train That Could" as an adult? When I would read this story to my kids I would try to instill its meaning (I think I can) to them. Without sounding ridiculous, the theme of this children's book is precisely on point for summoning up the focus needed to continue the recovery process. It is in this context that the words motivation and courage arise and they conjure up more than rote repetition of exercises day after day. The "more than rote repetition" is actually the mental focus needed to make the commitment active.

For me, the desire to give up was equal to the desire to succeed. I could feel the weight of hopelessness and failure. I was scared that no matter what I did it would still be fruitless. And the effort, day after day to persist continually, wore me down, eroding my resolve to be healthy. In order to mentally overcome the pain and stay motivated, I knew my courage and tenacity had to fully flower. The strength to persevere was not physical but an invisible interior quality. Recognizing that the draining of inner reserves continued through the siphon of pain, I realized it was an act of courage to remain strong and work the process through to completion. I discovered it was courage that built the mental strength necessary to pursue many of the activities I needed for my recovery.

An even larger realization was my discovery that simply living every moment and not quitting exemplifies courage in this new state.

Being involved in living is being a part of Nature and Nature is participating in my healing. She provides a never ending demonstration of death and rebirth, of motion and change, and of incandescent beauty in color. I had no idea how long it would take for Nature to complete her cycle and for me to accept what I had become. What I knew was that the manner in which I faced the new person staring back at me in the mirror, and my appreciation of him, is what would establish my courage.

I asked myself, do I want relief badly enough? Would I demand progress from myself day after day? If I answered "yes" to both questions, then I have agreed to vitalize myself enough to facilitate success. Only after I made this decision did the quality of "courage" become relevant.

Courage often exists when giving up is the easiest alternative. In the face of insurmountable odds, my desire for recovery drove the engine of hope. Because there was far more time each day when my feeling of hopelessness prevailed, overcoming this hopelessness was needed in order to insert success in its place.

For me, this hopelessness was a wash of gray, dense in oily thickness, appearing to limitlessly surround me. And like the post-snowstorm slush in the New York City streets, the dreary gray murkiness seemed to capture the desperation, as if anguish itself was being leeched from the soles of winter's booted feet. The vaguely understood gray fog, suspended in the air as if by antigravitational forces, invites me in. Yet once there I find myself blindly wandering, arms outstretched, searching for any solidity to support my weary body.

It makes no difference if the emotional courage to act is unearthed only in the face of blinding, insurmountable odds. Life presented me with my catastrophic event and now, under the weight of emotional upheaval, I can assume control over the tenor of how I will progress along my new life path. When I was neither fearful nor ashamed of my own courage I was able to accept the emotional vitality propelling me forward. This was a breakthrough in my healing.

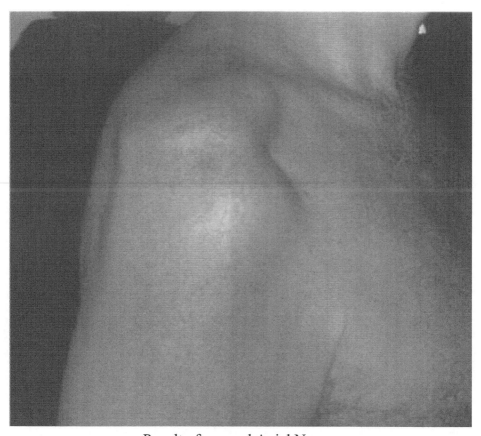
Result of severed Axial Nerve

MARC MAISLEN
SURGERY 07/11/2007: NERVE TRANSFER

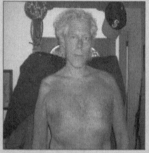

1. Photo of atrophied deltoid muscle

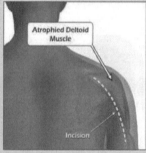

Atrophied Deltoid Muscle

Incision

2. Incision line and deltoid muscle

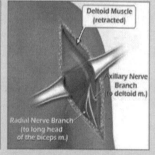

Deltoid Muscle (retracted)

Axillary Nerve Branch (to deltoid m.)

Radial Nerve Branch (to long head of the biceps m.)

3. Innervation of the deltoid muscle

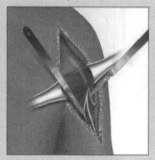

4. Transection of the nerves

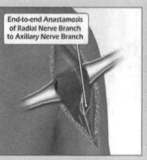

End-to-end Anastamosis of Radial Nerve Branch to Axillary Nerve Branch

5. Anastamosis of the nerve ends

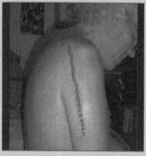

6. Post-op photo of surgical incision

Chapter Nineteen

THE DAILY GRIND

My recollection on the Work:

"I was a Spin Cycle instructor, teaching 3-4 classes a week, and now I'm on the stationary bike with resistance at 1 and I can't pedal for 20 minutes. I can barely hold onto the handlebars because of my right arm. I feel inadequate and my withered leg is a pathetic sight."

* * * *

"A man can only do what he can do. But if he does that each day he can sleep at night and do it again the next day."
- Albert Schweitzer –

* * * *

"I don't want you to be wonderful tomorrow. I just want you to be better than you are today."
- Paul J. Curtis –

When I would direct a project I would assign tasks to be completed by others: lighting design, costume execution or articles to be written. Suddenly there was nobody other than myself who was going to put in the hours of concentrated effort which hopefully would result in the completed task: my recovery. While there are many contributing specialists, they can only manipulate my body for brief, allotted periods of time. The remaining work rests on my shoulders and is up to me to do.

In the beginning of my recovery, physical therapy appointments lasted one hour twice a week. I looked forward to seeing my therapists, not only for the work itself but also because I was getting out of the house and becoming active in the world. Before the collision my old self stepped into the world each morning when I went to my job. After the crash my new self had a new job: working on my recovery.

The key component in achieving the most complete recovery was my commitment to do the necessary individual work to maximize my strength and flexibility, and to improve whatever deficits my injury had left me with. Quite a mouthful but these were the hurdles for me to overcome. The specific rehabilitation work was directed by therapists who instructed me on what exercises were designed for my recovery. These instructions shifted in scope and intensity as I improved. No sooner did I achieve a level of comfort in my exercise regime than a more difficult exercise was added. This, I discovered was how physical therapy works.

I did not give up. I did not lose hope. I approached each of these additional exercises and new plateaus as ever increasing heights along the mountain of recovery. I gave fresh energy to each of these new challenges. I gave myself the right to take my time with recovery but never deceived myself into thinking I was working hard when I was taking it easy. At the same time, I never deceived myself into believing that this process was simple when my inner self knew full well that this journey was conceivably the most difficult challenge I had ever tackled.

From out of the dark and into reality I see there are still many people in rehab. I am not alone. I am in the midst of a variety of focused people struggling with their disabilities. I breathe in the familiarity. I exhale tension. I breathe in the sense of family amongst the injured. I see many of the same faces. I am greeted by someone. We have seen each other before and I smile. I had difficulty getting up and out today. I breathe in strengthening energy. I am tired and not quite on top of it. I don't really want to work today. I am distracted and not motivated. I breathe in watching others work.

During hospital or office sessions, my therapists helped motivate me with positive words of encouragement. However, when I was at home sitting in front of the television knowing that my rehab required me to flex and release my hand ten times (and repeat it three times), the onus of exercising was squarely upon me. At home there was no professional who was being paid to inspire me. In fact, this was a solo performance in which no one else was present to remind me what exercises were required. It was during these solitary hours that I became fundamentally stronger because the strength I gained was not limited to the physical, but included the mental. By inspiring myself to action, I patted myself on the back, congratulated myself for a job well done, and gained confidence that I was furthering my recovery.

From the onset of rehabilitation, my experience of the work I was doing was one of pain. I have yet to meet anyone who engages in workouts in the rehab gym who has said to me, "this is the easiest thing I've done" or "what a snap." Rather, the consensus is that the work done in rehab is "medicine" and one that leaves an unpleasant taste.

Again, this irony of yet more pain arose for me. I had already been through an excruciatingly painful experience resulting in traumatic injury. Surviving it was the first hurdle. Then, in order to function as best as possible, I had to go through rehab and experience yet more pain during the recovery process. The irony of having to go through an extended period of pain during recovery after having already gone through horrendous pain during the trauma itself was almost too much for me to bear. At these times I experienced overwhelming moments of despair which triggered intense feelings of suicide. These feelings had to be moved through and released in order for me to go on. The irony of more pain to eliminate pain is the crossroad where committing to hopefulness and fighting the demons of suicide intersect.

There came a time when I found myself at that crossroads. I could no longer kid or deceive myself. The lure of giving up was seductive. Could I maintain a gung-ho attitude over an extended period of time? Where to turn? What to do? I had to persevere.

In the harsh light of reality I breathe in and look at myself in the mirror. Is there any obvious change? I breathe in strength and hopefulness. I breathe out any idea of pain. I see my body as clay that is being molded by me. I see the clay as being formed and reformed as an even stronger structure than before. I breathe in the small changes. I exhale the slowness of the process. I inhale my ability to build my body. I breathe out the need for immediate satisfaction. I look at myself and smile. I am stronger than last month.

The recovery process is similar to earning a college degree. After the first year or two of study I am wiser than when I began but I am also aware enough to know I have a long way to go before finishing. Do I still want the degree? Will I study for the final exams? Will I show up at class prepared and willing to participate? Do I want to challenge myself so that the results are meaningful? I want to answer 'yes' to these questions. I want to recover.

Participating in this recovery process is a true test of my character and could well be the hardest challenge I have ever worked through. In rehab I witnessed men and women who were neither athletes nor dancers vigorously work through their injuries with such passion and focus that their actions were an inspiration to me. Mary, a woman who had a prosthetic foot, was one of these people. Not only were her exercises vigorous but when she showed me her new foot I was moved by how she personally related to it and how she integrated her foot into her life making it her own. She was working hard and giving herself kudos for continuing to live a productive life. She was a great inspiration to me; a person who truly embodied the principle "I can."

The truth is that regardless of what age recovery is needed, it is never too late to confidently move through the minefield of difficult physical work. Once I was able to objectively evaluate the progress and results of my hard work, I was more effective in directing my energy into the positive and hopeful aspects of recovery.

When I met Mike, 62 years old and living in the rehab center, he was easily working on his lats while seated. I also sat, working on my leg with a simple leg raise. I leaned forward, cringing while raising my leg. He turned to me and said, "sit up and concentrate," which I did. When I jokingly said, "it's easy for you to say," he said, "Not really. My back is broken in multiple places." I felt so stupid and ashamed. After apologizing to him we spoke at length. His attitude that he was not asking for special treatment or sympathy deeply inspired me. Much worse off than me, he did not back down from life, so how could I? A powerful significant lesson learned.

Since adopting a recovery plan was new to me, the initial learning process was how these types of exercise programs work and which ones would be most effective for me. Most exercise regimens are designed to be repeated for a prescribed period of time; then another exercise takes its place. An alternative program has an exercise being repeatedly performed but with ever-increasing weights or resistance added. What I found most advantageous was a balance, a combination of both these types of exercise programs to achieve maximum results.

The key factor in either of these programs is in recognizing the success achieved. It was imperative for me to acknowledge the progress made over a period of time; a month being a reasonable time frame. This acknowledgement was crucial in my maintaining a positive and hopeful mental attitude. It also enabled me to quantify the positive changes I made as a result of my work. I was learning to be objective about my progress, whether it was greater stretch in my damaged muscles or the degree of motion in my rebuilt joints.

Not every day qualified as a big step forward. Quite the opposite! At the conclusion of most work sessions the result was not a recognizable major change. Rather, minor changes accrued every day ultimately leading to results over time. Patience was needed. When I was able to congratulate myself for my daily efforts, I was then allowing myself to recognize my incremental progress. And over time I was able to see the difference in strength, stretch and mobility.

Staying True to Myself

The mind is a complicated and tricky part of ourselves. On one hand we can deceive or convince ourselves that something is right even in the face of the opposite being true. On the other hand, we can also disengage the mind when it is trying to overwhelm us with negativity or pain. In the beginning of an enormous task it feels so much easier to give up and fold under the pressure. This is especially true when there is no guarantee that the task will be successful. In the long run, however, this path of least resistance might not produce the desired result.

What this means is if I shirk my responsibilities in doing my exercises I might feel more relaxed in that moment, but down the road I will likely be unable to achieve my goals of walking or using my arm. I must convince my mind that the short-term discomfort in struggling through the program of exercises is worth suffering through in order to achieve the possible result of enhanced physical ability. This is especially difficult because there often is not an immediately impressive result in doing the exercise program.

By adopting, integrating, and understanding the ever-shifting balance of excitement of the new versus the drudgery of the work and stretching the limits of what is possible versus the conservatism of what is safe, a neutral point must be reached. I strived to embody this new state of being which acknowledges the downside (the inability to walk) along with the pain of progress, and then counterbalances this by projecting and reinforcing a more healthy reality (actually walking).

Chapter Twenty

WORKING WITH ENERGY

My recollection on Performing:

"My therapist tells me I might be able to walk without limping. I see myself when I was dancing at the Delacorte Theatre and performing at Town Hall and Lincoln Center in New York City. I am retreating into my mind but I don't want to get lost there."

For most people there is a natural ebb and flow of energy levels during the course of a day. Eating healthy meals, having sufficient sleep and regularly exercising all contribute to creating and maintaining usable energy. After a traumatic event these patterns are disrupted.

Physical Energy

My former self drove my physical body around and through whatever obstacles arose during the course of a day. For example, if time was short and I needed to hustle through the aisles of the supermarket, my body responded appropriately: my legs moved faster and my heart rate increased. I had confidence that my body's response to the task at hand was up to snuff. When cleaning my house, moving furniture to locate dust bunnies or carrying the vacuum cleaner up to the second floor, there was no physical problem. In my new state, these simple activities take much longer to finish or cannot be accomplished without someone else's assistance.

My physical energy levels became inconsistent. Where I once could power through an activity for an hour, I now had to completely stop after ten minutes. At first I did not understand what had happened to me. As my atrophied muscles rebounded close to their former strength I worried what was wrong with me. I feared I had become a weak person. Over time, I realized that my physical energy was simply being siphoned off, redirected subconsciously, to the body parts that required healing; and there were many.

The repair to damaged bones, muscles, tissues and nerves requires attention twenty-four hours a day, seven days a week. A single broken arm requires seven weeks to fully heal. This adds up to a thousand hours! In my case, the traumatic event impacted almost all my body systems. I was only beginning to accept how many hours, weeks, months and probably years it would take for sufficient physical energy to be redirected so that healing would occur.

My physical rehabilitation was focused on building endurance and strength and gaining the power and determination to attempt activities over and over again. It was so strange going to the supermarket and having to rest after going up and down two aisles. I wanted to continue but did not have the strength. Eventually, by exercising more patience with the process than I imagined I possessed, my accessible physical energy incrementally increased to a near normal state.

I love cycling and for me 10-30 mile jaunts were normal. So as a life-long cyclist I assumed that the stationary bike would be a breeze. But this exercise demonstrated the terrible extent of my injuries as well as the degree of growth I was able to achieve. I began my biking rehab about eight weeks after the collision with a starting degree of difficulty at #2 out of 25. Imagine my surprise when I could not rotate my legs for more than five minutes. By the end of the month, after using the bike three times a week, my resistance level had increased to #4 and I could cycle for ten minutes. Continuing this procedure, I consistently improved until I reached difficulty #12 with non-stop cycling for twenty minutes. This took one year. Although I was not out on the open road and I still needed to use the recumbent bike, I was actually cycling.

Mental Energy

My former self maintained a steady stream of thoughts, weighing right and wrong, analyzing data, and clarifying and classifying a variety of input in order to determine correct courses of action.

Because of my brain injury, for well over a year, my new self did not possess the steady concentration required to make lucid decisions. Whether the brain is hyperactive or sluggish and wobbly, neither of these states is conducive to logical linear thinking. I was experiencing both. A ship on a calm sea allows the passengers to enjoy the journey and view miles of gorgeous ocean. However, if the seas are choppy and enormous waves are crashing against the ship, visual acuity is limited and motion can make the passengers sea sick.

Even more problematic was the fact that I was accustomed to using my intelligence, my brain power to solve problems. I thrived on being able to analyze an issue, gather information about it and make decisions I could stand behind. Suddenly I felt abandoned. I could not rely on my orderly intelligence to clarify what was happening. I needed to constantly try to illuminate my own confusion.

Mental energy relies, to a large extent, on the ability to concentrate. This focus is the steadiness required to determine what is needed, how to go about getting it, and correctly choosing the method of achieving the goal. My mental energy could no longer sustain these thoughts to a satisfactory conclusion. Like a slow leaking tire, when I needed to roll all I had was a flat. Did my injury suddenly make me stupid? Was I so disconnected that I no longer cared about what happened? Again, not at all. Rather, some force was causing my mental energy to be disrupted, impeding the flow of ideas. I realized this unseen force was pain.

Part of my diminished problem solving skills was because when pain is constant, the nagging discomfort erodes the ability to maintain concentration. When pain is present it acts like a vampire, robbing energy from the system and causing a weakening of the mind's focus.

In my moments of clarity I wondered whether it was possible to stabilize this rollercoaster ride. And if pain relief drugs are employed, as in the vast majority of cases where a traumatic event has occurred, how do they affect one's mental state?

Shattered

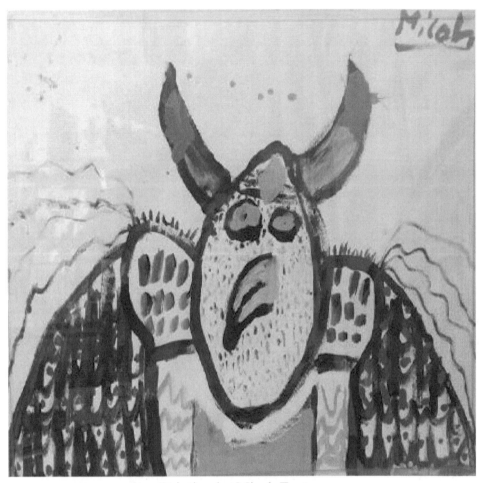

Painting by Micah Eastman

Chapter Twenty-One

MEDICATION AND WITHDRAWAL

My recollection on Control:

"I'm home in bed. The pain is keeping me awake. No meds for three more hours. All I really want to do is go dancing, clubbing, or even late night eating. I can't do this. I want to scream in frustration. I can't remember the last time I was fun to be around."

My first physical therapist, while I was still hospitalized, insisted I take pain medication an hour prior to arriving at my session because I was grunting too loudly and disturbing other patients. She was harsh with me but I quickly understood the effect of pain medication was to enable me to make a legitimate effort at executing the rehab exercises. If I was unable to perform these exercises I would ultimately have a seriously diminished ability to recover from my injuries.

Right from the outset I knew what performing the exercises meant. When I used to rehearse for hours, after repeating the same movement phrase, I would make many slight corrections during the rehearsal process. When I performed the work, all my heart and soul was infused in it. Each movement, each extension, each idea had the totality of my being finding expression. With an audience of one, my rehab exercises took on the same quality as performance.

Unlike dancing freely, rehab needed a boost; a shot in the arm so to speak. I quickly came to the conclusion that pain medication was this useful mode of treatment. Western science has spent countless sums of money in developing medications for a wide range of ills. Whether taking medication for depression, allergies or pain, we are putting our faith in the fact that a substance exists designed to alleviate specific symptoms. In my case, the meds short circuited the registration of pain in my brain so I would not suffer the full extent of it.

When we have massive bone or internal injuries, the pain does not subside overnight. My pain was relentless, seldom dipping below seven or eight on a scale of ten. Without the use of pain medication my life would have been miserable and far too unbearable for me to make steady improvement.

While acknowledging that pain medication is useful, I also recognized its enormous down side: the most effective pain medications have addictive properties. These meds are generally morphine based or composed of a narcotic that is addictive. It is the narcotic properties that kill the pain. At the end of my therapy or when I was well enough to handle a moderate level of pain, I knew the next vital hurdle for me clear was to wean off the pain medication.

I have become acutely aware of the various gradations of pain. When I went to the hospital for follow-up exams, I was always asked to rate the level of pain I was experiencing. I was thrilled that, over time, I saw my pain level diminishing. But I also recognized after a year of medication, the low end of pain never reduced to zero. There was always a steady pain percolating under the surface of consciousness arising at random points during the day. Pain's unwelcome intrusion became more and more disturbing to me because it never relented.

My Recollection on Sleep:

"I wake up because I hear sounds. The sound is getting louder. I wake up and realize that I am making the sound. I am moaning. I am in pain. I am deeply moaning. I know I am in my bed but there is no comfort. The pain is not going away."

Another level of challenge arose when it became obvious that the pain was not disappearing. Would the level of pain never fall below a tolerable point? Would there be a never-ending necessity for the administration of pain killers? If so, this was an unacceptable solution for me.

While pain killers are serving the purpose of pain reduction, dependency is the result. This dependency has its own problems. First, the mind does not think as clearly when in a drug induced state. And second, when we are ready to stop the medication we have to experience the discomfort of withdrawal. In order to free oneself from pain medication it is necessary to methodically reduce the daily dosage of the medication until the body no longer has a craving for it.

Reducing pain medication entails overcoming two hurdles: psychologically agreeing to eliminate the dependency on medication; and, physically going through pain. Yes, another irony of recovery. In order to free oneself from dependency on pain medication the withdrawal process produces pain in the body.

Often, after a traumatic event, the injured person regularly ingests pain medication for a period of time; in my case for about a year and a half. What occurs on a daily basis is that without thinking about pain but also without taking any medication, a feeling of pain will suddenly arise. If bones are healing, nerves are still growing, or if the muscles have atrophied and need to be stretched and strengthened, the body, not the mind will give a signal which we experience as pain. Since the medication produces a dependency on it, if we do not take the pill or if we reduce the dosage of the pill, the body will cry out for more. The body is relying on this dosage to maintain the status quo. The body is demanding a degree of relief so it does not experience pain.

The point where this experience of pain becomes clouded is during the withdrawal process. Under a doctor's supervision it will be agreed upon it is time to wean off the medication. However, the body is not agreeing to this; the doctor and patient are making this pact. The body is heedless of the program. The body wants to continue to be pain free and have a sense of relief from the injuries. But when we begin this weaning process it is because the body, in reality, is no longer in such dire need of chemical intervention. The body is far enough along in the healing process that it no longer faces the same degree of pain. What the body is now experiencing is the desire to feel "smooth." Even though there is not the debilitating pain, the body wants the smoothness.

What is this smoothness? In my previous life I might have become agitated at something and by breathing and relaxing felt normal again. That was my daily smoothness. Most of us do not take drugs in order to feel smooth. I know I didn't. I dealt with agitation with the knowledge that in a short time I would return to a moderate level of balance. But in this new life which includes a dependency, I have inserted a chemical to quickly and artificially balance my body. During the extreme pain stage this was necessary, worthwhile and healthy. But at this new stage, the agitation of the body is not a manifestation of pain or our injuries. It is a manifestation of the body itself as if it was a petulant child yelling, "I want this; I want my meds." And the body keeps screaming that it wants it. If I am confused about what is happening, I will believe I am still in pain. But with my attention on withdrawal I can more clearly recognize that it is my body that is independently yelling for pain killers.

This screaming is not a function of the pain from my car crash or rehabilitation. It is the child wanting another piece of cake or demanding more ice cream. I must rely upon my adult self to inform the child it cannot have what it wants right now. This is the tough love I had to impose on myself. This is my higher Self wanting to be healthy and bargaining with the child that it can have a little chocolate but not the entire chocolate bar. If the child was overweight but accustomed to eating a bag of potato chips every day I would have to lower the portion of chips to get the child back to its healthy weight. Withdrawal is the same program. By eliminating portions of pain killers a little at a time, eventually the need for any pain killers will disappear.

Again, the irony that I had to experience more pain to eliminate the dependency on pain killers was horrible to face. Yet I knew that relying on pain killers was not the answer. I wanted off them as soon as possible, therefore, I had to face this path of withdrawal with determination.

Mental Effect

We do not think as clearly when we are on pain killers as when we are free from medication. Even though the body is feeling more mellow and so the mind is filled with less static, the flow of ideas, the ability to truly concentrate and persevere, and the capacity to communicate in a focused fashion are all diminished.

For example, when watching a movie I would be unable to register the continuing story line. Minutes would pass when my brain would seemingly be asleep. Similarly, when watching a baseball game on TV I would find I did not know what inning was being played. Much worse, however, was when I would have an idea, whether creative or practical, and I could not completely flesh it out. For example, I would have an image of a performer touching his heart and reaching up but I would not see the subsequent image, the next movement flowing out, after the performer's reach. Or I would want grilled fish for dinner but I did not have the follow-up thought of what marinade to use; or I would totally forget what vegetable went best with the fish.

It may appear that thinking is less agitated when smoothed out by pain killers. The truth is, thinking while on pain killers is sluggish because thoughts are moving through a muddier environment. The chemical is producing a cloudier space in the brain which affects all mental activity. There is an unnatural dampening of the thought processes. Whether this produces less verbal clarity, a lessened ability to laugh, or even more difficulty in following multiple lines of thought, the administering of pain killers has this subtle, and often not so subtle, impact on the brain.

Pain Tolerance

This mental/emotional aspect of withdrawal is directly tied to the psychological impact of weaning off pain killers. While this does not appear logical given that pain is physically felt, I am referring to withdrawal in terms of a psychological state. The following explanation will make this clearer.

During withdrawal the body is responding in an agonizing way. The best way to describe this is that you are feeling as if your body is turning inside out; or that your insides are pushing against your skin from the inside, trying to get out. This is where the physical pain is experienced. However, this pain is not real. This pain is not associated with your injuries. This pain is directly related to withdrawal symptoms. The biggest hurdle to overcome in this process is having the psychological fortitude to withstand the degree of discomfort experienced. The feeling of the body turning inside out is no minor event. Without the psychological strength to deal with this, it could break a person's spirit or drive them back to taking meds to alleviate the discomfort. I struggled with this conflict every day during withdrawal. It was not pleasant.

The dream/reality is never more apparent as when I breathe in and try to exhale the pain. Each muscle, bone and skin is vibrating. I breathe in and out, panting. There is no localized pain. It is everywhere. I breathe in hope and relief. My body is desperately contracting with anxiety. I must breathe.

I found that taking a Tylenol is useful in reducing edginess, but it did not stop me from sitting and moaning for an hour. The first day of withdrawal was the most difficult, with the second day a bit less stressful. After I stabilized at the new, reduced level of medication for a week or two, the same miserable process began again when the doctor further reduced my dosage. I again felt the inside/out pain with an overwhelming degree of agitation. Although it was not an easy process, I knew it was imperative I fully re-engage my psychological brain functioning in order for this portion of my healing to be complete.

Pain tolerance during withdrawal has different qualities than pain tolerance during the height of injury recovery. During withdrawal the mind can and will play tricks on a person. The relentlessly pounding desire to take the meds to soothe the agitation makes normal functioning extremely difficult. Without constant attention, the mind can easily be swayed causing a breakdown in the determination to stop taking the medication. Remember that the agitation and apparent pain are part of the illusion of need. My body was craving the pain killers but my recovery from injury was not demanding the meds. This is a mind game that demanded my complete focus. I knew the agitation would pass. I knew I would progress through the distress of the moment and become free of the dependency on pain killers if I persevered. I was determined to do so.

What was it that allowed me to not give up and regress into dependency in this process? For me it was a simple anchor: counting time. When I took a reduced dose of oxycontin/oxycodone I would feel relief for 2 hours. Unfortunately, the next scheduled dose was 3-4 hours away. As my discomfort/withdrawal symptoms increased, I would look at the clock and say, "Only 3 more hours to go." Then when discomfort arose again, I would look at the clock and say, "Only 2 ½ more hours to go." This time check gave me the solid ground, the framework to envision when the discomfort would be over. Withdrawal takes time so seeing the end of the tunnel saw me through to the next dose and ultimately to the reduction of any symptoms at all. I had mastered it; I was free.

Sadly, the withdrawal process was the singularly most isolating experience I have ever gone through. No therapist, wife or friend could assist me. Perhaps, because of the extent of nerve damage I suffered in my hand, elbow, shoulder and hip I was more sensitive to the lack of pain relief formerly provided by the oxycontin, then oxycodone. All I know is that any support I received came from within because nothing helped illuminate the dark, bleak pit of withdrawal.

Since then, an over-the-counter medication that has been helpful with no apparent side effects has been Advil. I continue to take anywhere between six to sixteen Advils a day. My body is not free of pain but I am free of the dependency on opioids (pain killers). My body no longer screams for the addictive pain killers because I can take Advil to alleviate enough pain for me to function adequately. I know I am taking charge of my life because the pain killers are not controlling me or my mind.

Resources:

The Pain Relief Handbook : Self-Help Methods for Managing Pain by Chris Wells, Graham Nown, Chrissie Wells, Ronald Melzack
Overcoming Chronic Pain: A Self-Help Guide Using Cognitive Behavioral Techniques by Frances Cole, Hazel Howden-Leach, Helen Macdonald, Catherine Carus
How to Get Off Psychoactive Drugs Safely: There is Hope. There is a Solution by James Harper N.C. (Author), Jayson Austin N.C. (Contributor)

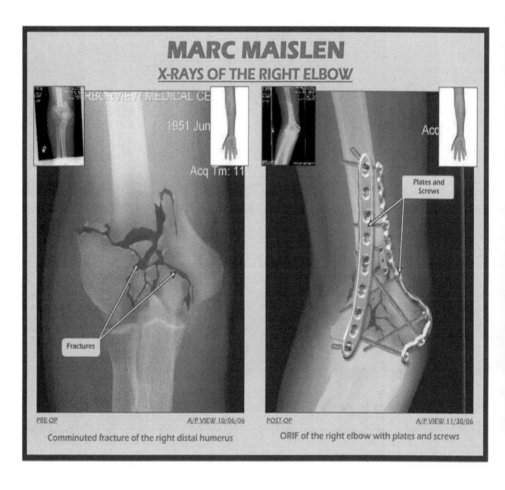

MARC MAISLEN

X-RAYS OF THE RIGHT ELBOW

PRE-OP — A/P VIEW 10/06/06
Comminuted fracture of the right distal humerus

POST-OP — A/P VIEW 11/30/06
ORIF of the right elbow with plates and screws

Chapter Twenty-Two

CONFRONTING TRUTH

My recollection on my leg Blood Clot:

"I can barely touch my lower leg. The pain is awful. After a month of complaining, the doctors finally agree to give me a sonogram. It is revealed that I have a blood clot in my leg. Now I have to give myself two shots a day for thirty days to dissolve the clot. I need to inject myself in the stomach morning and night. More crap to deal with. I really don't like needles."

* * * *

"Perhaps everything terrible is in its deepest being something helpless that wants help from us."
- Rainer Maria Rilke –

"There is no such thing as chance; and that which seems to us blind accident actually stems from the deepest source of all."
- Friedrich von Schiller -

The injury is the truth. The pain is the truth. The incapabilities are the truth. Who I once was is no longer the truth. This new, unrecognized self is the truth.

Out of the dark dream box I am feeling more in control. I look at my body. I try not to gasp but to breathe steadily. I breathe in and out feeling my lungs fill and release. This person cannot be me but the more I look at myself the more I realize this new person is me. I move the parts of my body I can. I breathe in, knowing that parts of me are strange and need to be learned again. I thought I was in control but I don't know how to control my new body. I feel fear, confusion and disconnection. I breathe again and as I relax and loosen my hold on these emotions I see these emotions do not have a death grip on me. I breathe and experience an even greater loosening of their stranglehold. I catch a glimpse of myself in a mirror. I breathe and smile. There I am. I am me.

It is extremely difficult to look at my new self as the truth, as who I am. Surely I am not this new, incapable person. Surely I am still the independent, self determined person I always was. Surely when I look in the mirror, the person looking back at me is the one I remember as myself. Yet, this is incorrect. How can this person looking back at myself be so alien, so unrecognizable?

I need to learn who this new person is. I need to stop listening to what my inner voice has been reaffirming, for my entire life, about who I am. I need to develop a sense that registers the new self that I am. This new person I call self is hearing sounds and words differently, seeing life and shadows from a fresh perspective, and feeling the highs and lows of random emotions that have the same surprising colorations as did the raging hormones of puberty.

The sooner I recognize, acknowledge and accept this new self, the more successful I can be in starting to rebuild and create my new life. I deserve an opportunity to uncover my newness.

When I stepped onto the stage in character, the foundation work in selecting the attributes, strengths and weaknesses of the character were of my choosing. The skill to select qualities and then highlight them in performance was built into my system. Years of repetition guaranteed a consistent result. By taking these same steps I employed in isolating my theatrical truth, locating and defining my new-found reality was crucial in becoming and inhabiting my newborn self.

Taking the time to focus on developing my character and believing in my worthiness is not selfish. It also makes no sense that my self esteem needs to be dictated by other peoples' prejudices and frailties. It does not have to be that way. I must first empower myself. Without attributing myself with merit there is no compelling reason to continue.

When my thoughts started to clear up, I had already been damaged, hospitalized and moved to a rehab facility. So after a month or two I had the clarity to project how long I'd be taking to get better. Since I'd broken bones when I was younger, I estimated that in a month or two I'd be healed. But when I talked to the doctors and was informed what the extent of my damages were, I slowly and painfully realized that a quick resolution into full use of my body was unrealistic. For example, when I was told I was not allowed to lift anything heavier than a pencil with my right arm and that my fingers couldn't bend for 6 months, I was stopped in my tracks. Then being told I needed Occupational Therapy to hopefully regain full movement, this mirror image of me was going to be a man I needed to get acquainted with.

In order to cleanse myself of old notions I must first recognize that the possibility of a different state can exist. I must perceive value in this difference or how can I make the sacrifices necessary to make the change? There can be no doubt that my self esteem will breathe or suffocate in response to my attention. To fully inspire this self worth, in the way the blossoming essence of Spring removes the quilt of Winter, is to understand myself. If I was to smother this awakening, it would only reinforce the gut-wrenching contraction that weakens me. I do not want that. I want to be awake.

It is vital to reiterate that believing in my worthiness is a value that adds to my character, my self. In addition, the cleansing shower of personal growth is not a forgotten dust-covered attribute of some vague aspect of my past. It, too, is real. I know my slate will never be wiped free of history but the palette can be refreshed so that the cooling, distinct flavors of life can be distinguished from the bitter residue of my pain.

Injury

The mind will recognize whatever input is run through the brain and senses. So on one level, the continuity from pre-injury to current injured state does not miss a beat. The Self knows that the organism is injured and proceeds accordingly. This was perfectly apparent when after my hip socket was rebuilt my body refused to walk on it. My Self knew this activity could not yet be performed.

The wonder of the new reality is when my eyes are closed, standing in front of the mirror. I breathe in and slowly exhale opening my eyes. I have glimpsed myself before but now I carefully look at myself. Nothing exists other than me and the mirror. I tune my mind into being a child; the innocence of youth. I have no expectations of what I will see; I will see what I am now. I breathe and smile at the knowledge that I am alive and seeing myself. I steadily breathe in and out. I am no longer in the dark. I am alive and in the light of a new me that is continuing to change. I breathe in my new self.

The neural networking in my brain has established my past pattern of functioning. The neural net, combined with my consciousness or desire to do an activity, sets up an expectation of normalcy and success. This normalcy is my pre-injury functioning factor. My mind wants to continue to repeat this. My mind wants to believe that this successful way of functioning will continue uninterrupted and with equally positive results. The more difficult reality to come to terms with is that my prior years of activity can no longer predictably produce the same results.

What is more problematic is that I want to believe this deception of the mind. Why wouldn't I? This deception preserves the picture of health and normalcy. However, since the only way I will be able to approach the ability to function normally again is by first acknowledging the limitations I need to overcome, I have to let go of this deception, the resistance to "what is." The initial recognition of the injury is an enormously difficult hurdle to overcome.

When people would visit me shortly after my car crash they would ask "how are you?" and I would respond "fine." On one level I did not want them to pity me after my having told them the truth, but on a deeper level I was in denial. The truth was that I was not fine. I did not feel comfortable, social, cheerful, ready to share, excited, concentrated, or in any way good. I was in pain. The idea of saying I was fine did not result in me being fine; it only continued the deception by denying the truth of my new self.

Compassion

Why does my mind want to persist in thinking all is well? Why do I hold onto the past? Why does it feel like my memory of what existed before my life-changing event is more important than what is happening right now?

In the past, I never wanted to appear weak, knowing that most people are raised to see others who are injured, crippled, or challenged in any number of ways as objects of pity, essentially less than whole. It was simpler to intellectually address the issues of physically and mentally challenged people. I rarely allowed their challenges to touch my heart. This did not present a problem since our culture teaches a mistrust and fear of disability as opposed to an awakening into compassion for others. I am different now.

In the new reality of my becoming whole I am relaxing watching TV. My favorite program is on. I shift my position so that I don't feel as much pain. I breathe and relax. A commercial comes on asking people to send money to help children with disabilities. The TV shows these kids. I want to turn away. My old self wants to disregard this. I keep staring at the TV. My eyes fill up with tears. I don't know these kids but I feel for them. My heart feels like it is up in my throat. I feel sadness and another feeling: compassion. I breathe and nod with understanding. I am not alone in this new world of mine. I wipe my eyes and softly smile

The moment of my incapability was like a blinding light bursting into my brain, illuminating a worst case scenario. But this is not a worst case scenario at all. Rather, it is the truth of living on the other side of the veil, the side I never believed would be my home. Living on this other side, the side where people stare at me and wonder what happened to me and wonder what is wrong with me and feel sorry for me, this side is incapable of functioning in the old way of life. Nevertheless, this side is fully capable in a different and unexpected way; this side is my new truth.

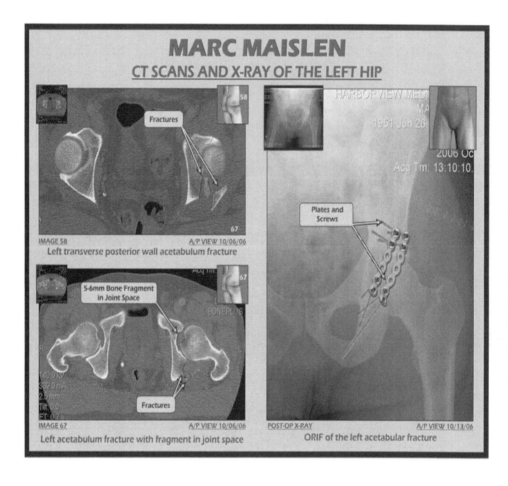

MARC MAISLEN
CT SCANS AND X-RAY OF THE LEFT HIP

Fractures

IMAGE 58   A/P VIEW 10/06/06
Left transverse posterior wall acetabulum fracture

5-6mm Bone Fragment in Joint Space

Fractures

IMAGE 67   A/P VIEW 10/06/06
Left acetabulum fracture with fragment in joint space

Plates and Screws

POST-OP X-RAY   A/P VIEW 10/13/06
ORIF of the left acetabular fracture

Chapter Twenty-Three

WHAT IS PROGRESS?

My recollection on being photographed:

"I would look in the mirror after my shower. But I wasn't really looking and seeing. Having my picture taken froze my image. The red, swollen, stapled, scarred body was mine. I need to love me."

The most important aspect in evaluating my progress was being kind to myself. I knew the one thing I should not do was to harshly judge my failures. An essential element in my steady recovery was to persevere, especially when I thought I was not doing enough. I learned that in working on many goals, whether large or small, I was worthy of the progress I was making.

No matter how altered and unrecognizable my new self appeared to me, when I judged myself negatively it wasted potentially positive energy. I had to remind myself to consider how much better off I would be if the time spent on being harsh and critical of my self was channeled into being positive and helpful. It is no surprise that self directing positivity is easier said than done.

Additionally, who is determining what progress represents? When I could barely shuffle along and my surgeon told me the operation was a success, this was progress to him. But I needed to actually walk before I was willing to agree that this was progress.

Progress can be broken down into physical and emotional as well. It is so much easier to calibrate physical progress since increasing the load of weights or the number of repetitions is clearly evident. This progress is also very satisfying. I'm lifting more weights so my arm is getting stronger.

Emotional progress is much more elusive. How was I able to

quantify that my sadness was lessening? Or my depression wasn't as bleak? Or that my loneliness and detachment was not permanent? There was no chart to track this progress. The dark form of emotions cast shadows at unexpected moments and there is very little substance to grab hold of.

Emotional progress is also subjective and whether a psychotherapist is involved to help you through difficult times or whether meditation is employed to calm, center and clarify self, addressing this fragile aspect of who you are is crucial for recovery. A smile while making fun of yourself or not getting angry when having problems standing without assistance are positive markers along the road of emotional recovery.

I had to be alert, mindful, patient and relentless in both being aware of emotional outbursts and in breathing through and finding ways to defuse these eruptions. This was not a simple task.

I knew I truly wanted a constructive result. One of the simplest devices I used for achieving this positive outcome was to take a moment when I was feeling the lack of progress or incapacity and then, while taking a breath, state to myself that each small step was adding up to a larger movement. By allowing myself to see and accept the bigger picture, that there is room for change and growth, I felt an immediate sense of release and relaxation.

Judgment is like an inchworm feeding on the food of hope. With such an insatiable appetite one must be careful not to focus on negative self-judgment. After a traumatic event, being in pain, not knowing what the future holds and being dependent on medication, the door is wide open for negative judgment. I told myself it was important not to deny these negative truths but rather to accept them as temporary states of being. My personal power grew with the knowledge that these states can be shifted over time into a more functional and healthier sense of self.

Resources:

The Tibetan Art of Positive Thinking: Skillful Thought for Successful
Living by Christopher Hansard
Positive Affirmations: 92 Affirmations That Apply Positive Quotes And
Positive Words To Banish Negative Thinking by Gary Vurnum

Chapter Twenty-Four

PERCEPTION OF OTHERS

Recollection from Bedroom:

"This is it. I am what I've seen in others. I don't want anyone to see me like this. I want to disappear. This is not me. This cannot be me."

* * * *

"I'm rounding the corner from anything that's real
I'm across the road from hope
I'm under a bridge in a rip tide
That's taken everything I call my own
One step closer to knowing...
One step closer to knowing..."
- U2 -

Prior to my traumatic life-changing event I had adopted roles in my life that identified me as a productive, responsible and active member of society. I generally knew who I was and I was usually seen this way by others.

As a post-trauma survivor I am no longer viewed in this optimistic way. But more distressing is when people make negative judgmental comparisons. For example, others might say, "He was once so good looking" or "He was such a terrific tennis player" or "I used to be able to listen to him for hours." Though these statements are probably true, the underlying emotional tone of these observations is generally one of pity or of feeling sorry for me. Imagine my surprise when I experienced people unable to look me in the eye when I was in a wheelchair, when they noticed my scars or when I could not move a limb properly.

These examples are basically emotionally damaging, but over time another issue arises out of this negative feedback which compounds the problem. What arose for me was I began to take in this feedback and feel negatively about myself. I adopted these negative attributes as if they were mine. Ultimately, I realized that feeling sorry for myself or being embarrassed about my new condition is far worse than what another person is saying about me.

This in no way removes my sadness about my loss of ability or how upset I am about the way I now look. This is about the attitude attached to that judgment. Some people who are not living the same reality as I, are quick to assume I am not really that bad off or that I am faking my condition in order to gain sympathy. Other people are overly sympathetic, bending over backwards to mask their own feeling of discomfort with my condition.

Rather than wasting my energy getting mad at other people, it is vital for my mental health that I disregard everyone else's judgment about me and address my own challenges.

The key to disregarding others' judgment was my repeated visits to the orthopedic center at the hospital. It was there, as I awaited being x-rayed every 2-4 weeks, that I sat next to, conversed with and simply viewed men, women and children in the waiting area. Over half these people were injured or disfigured far worse than I. By looking at how I was judging others, I came around full circle, seeing how I was actually judging myself. Only then was I able to free myself.

Immersed in the reality of life I breathe in the sunshine. I feel the handle of my cane and trust the support the shaft gives me. I breathe in and out, calming myself as I enter the mall. There is a whirlwind of motion. I breathe in and out as I walk into the flow. Some people look at me, at my limp; others give me a wide berth. I breathe. I am in the world. I am just another person shopping. I smile and nod in acceptance.

PART IV
COMING INTO THE LIGHT

Chapter Twenty-Five

CHARTING THE UNKNOWN

Recollection from Hospital Bed:

"I find I am in a waking dream. There are recognizable avenues but no streets to turn into. Trapped, my eyes roll upward in search of an escape. There is a thin band of light high above a shadowy alley. Is this real or an illusion? Feeling desperate I assume this must be the way out. Or is it?"

* * * *

"Man doesn't choose the moment.
The moment chooses the man."
- Anonymous -

Just when I thought I knew it all, one thing became clear. Activities, plans, apparent realities or ideas of truth and justice I had prior to the collision vanished in less than one second. Having the experience that my life could be snuffed out so quickly before my brain could comprehend what was going on was an outrageous concept. In that moment, my path was inexorably altered; the railroad switch was thrown and I was diverted onto an unknown track. What I once believed to be important became secondary and the familiar became unrecognizable. What I had imagined my life's purpose to be was forever altered.

The perspective that I once perceived as familiar was replaced by the singular purpose of regaining my balance in this ever-shifting landscape. The pleasure of floating in a lazy drifting creek was replaced by fighting to survive in a torrent of water. The Earth became so unstable that what I once counted on as solid ground transmuted itself into a soft mire dotted with bottomless sinkholes. Where I once believed I was fearless, I was now face to face with my fear which was previously masked in bravado. I was forced to re-examine many of my behaviors which once came naturally to me. My courage to take action was redefined into something much simpler and also infinitely more difficult: the courage to BE.

I was forced to view my life frame by frame, slowing down the movie so I could see, touch and savor the sacredness of Now. While this can be looked at as a philosophical ideal, the moments after my devastating event truly embodied this principle. Philosophy can give a framework of ideas around a core truth but, when I was "dead," there was no philosophy to grasp. And, when I "awoke," the philosophies no longer had the power to move me into a way of living life.

My collision involved another person as well as myself. He was not physically injured but his life was turned upside down, just like mine, due to vehicular assault charges and devastating criminal court appearances. Without my presence in the path of his truck he would not have had the opportunity to clean up his life. Similarly, without his truck appearing out of nowhere and crushing me, I would not have had the opportunity to open up to a different experience of patience, compassion and understanding. But this was not a conscious choice since my everyday mind did not select a particular truck to converge with. It was my deep unconscious mind that recognized the moment of opportunity and chose to put me in harm's way creating a devastating collision. Whether I subsequently made a new conscious choice to exercise my body, mind and heart in a different way than I had in the past, was up to me.

When I stopped blaming another person for what had happened to me, identifying myself as a "victim," and gently replaced "blame" with "choice," (no matter how outrageous this appears), another beacon of possibility illuminating the darkness opened up. I believe I made the choice to participate in a life-altering, horrendously painful car crash. Afterward, by recognizing this choice on my path and (finally) consciously accepting it, I was then able to more quickly make intelligent, sensitive adjustments in order to acknowledge myself and make my new life work.

The fact that life was new, fresh, unexpected and vibrant was the gift given to me. The truth of me as survivor was no longer about ideas, but rather about actuality. The moment became filled with what is; not a step toward some elusive future. I was brought face to face with the reality of my existence as it unfolded in front of me. That positive aspect of reality, what some might call God's plan, was the most valuable lesson I learned because of my near catastrophic crash. I learned there is only the Eternal Now.

Viewing the frames of my life was often confusing and having crushed bones did not make any sense. I had a strong image of a functioning body while watching Arnold Schwartzenegger in "Total Recall" run through the airport x-ray machine. I even remember the innocuous skeleton hanging in the corner of the science class room as waves of us marched past it during the course of the year; a complete set of bones. To connect what we look like underneath the skin, in motion, stimulates the mind into wondering how in the world this all stays together.

It is understandable that the image of having crushed bones is totally abstract for most people. Unfortunately for me, it was something I was forced to confront after my life was redirected because of another person's thoughtless actions.

Thank goodness there was far too much noise during my collision for me to hear so many of my bones breaking. But imagine the image of handling a lead pencil. The lead is like bone marrow; too soft to be a factor. Grab both ends of the pencil and bend. There is flexibility as the wood grudgingly gives in to the pressure being exerted upon it. The resistance of the wood returns the pencil to its original shape not dissimilar to our bones flexing and realigning themselves. Exert more pressure by placing your thumbs at the mid-length point of the pencil while bending it. Suddenly the pencil will snap in half, emitting a percussive crack at the moment of breaking. This single sound happened to me twenty five years ago as I was teaching a movement class. I stepped awkwardly on my right foot, and as it rolled over I heard the unmistakable crack of my foot breaking. The students around me also heard the sound and visibly paled when I said, "I just broke my foot." The sensation of my own bones breaking is far more potent than the simple similarity to the sound of a pencil snapping.

The sensation of my body breaking is unlike anything I have ever experienced. A kiss may be indescribable but breaking bones is both indescribable and bizarre. In the same way I once took for granted the stability of the Earth until I was standing on rolling, undulating ground in Seattle's largest earthquake in fifty years, I never doubted the strength and steadiness of my skeletal system until it proved fallible after all.

One aspect of when a bone breaks is the sense of disbelief. For example, when I am with someone and my stomach growls but I do not know whether it is my stomach or theirs, I am momentarily confused, albeit with the attendant humor, as to where exactly the source of the growl is originating. Like cocking the head to help locate whose stomach is growling, turning to look at the affected/broken body part is a natural reaction. The mind even plays a trick in changing disbelief to an "I hope not" moment. This initial denial where no external physical evidence exists supporting what the sound of bone snapping has done to the body is part of the uncomfortable feeling.

At that moment of breaking when my linear brain goes "uh oh," the broken body parts begin to register pain and my perceptions are inextricably altered as adrenaline floods through every cell in my body. But in the seconds before this protective mechanism consumes me and registers pain in real time, there is a sickening sensation, like finding yourself in free fall after jumping off the high diving board. There is the sense of inevitability, of no going back. What was regarded as solid ground a moment before is now questionable.

If I am breaking, does that mean I am breakable? Obviously it does! What follows is that I am not indestructible; I am vulnerable. Does breaking mean total inability to be repaired; or is breaking a simple bump in the road, soon to be planed, paved and ready to be sped across better than ever before? Does breaking mean one clean, efficient rupture in the continuity or, is this breaking a total shattering of what existed before?

When I am feeling the inescapable reality that my body is broken, the weight of my destiny presses down on me like the ever increasing pressure of water as one swims deeper and deeper. Even though I feel like throwing my arms up in the air and yelling "enough is enough!" I know that there is no going back. I am terribly confused by the inevitability of my fate. I tell myself that perhaps having had broken bones earlier in my life was merely the preparation for my current misfortune.

The Changing Landscape

Broken bones are not the only changes forced upon me. Another change is that sometimes as my mind wanders I wonder whether this wandering is a product of my new lack of consistent concentration due to my brain injury. Where my old self wanted to be focused and concentrated on whatever I desired, now my desires appear to take a back seat to what actually is. Perhaps being dis-abled is in reality a way of moving into being en-abled. It's exciting to sense so much more to be discovered.

Like the thrilling moments when I first learned the rules of chess or board games, discovering a deep desire for awareness, love, expansion and enlightenment was mind-blowing. Just having the knowledge of this desire TO BE was an integral part of revealing a greater truth in the game of life.

If, as Joni Mitchell sang, "we go round and round and round in the circle game," then there have been many circles I have traversed in my life. These circles, by definition, have neither a beginning nor an end yet they appear as different paths, like securing a job or starting a family. And each has a life of its own. I wondered if having a life-changing event makes these separate circles disappear? Does a single, powerful event break the multitude of circles? Does this event demonstrate that each circle is made up of a series of connected points (events) as well as any number of flowing arcs? And further, are we really on one continuous circle, where life itself highlights the journey in the infinite number of possible points (events) and flowing arcs? If this is true, do we actually shape the circle by our participation in the journey or is everything predestined and revealed at the precise moment of intention? Are we even in control of this intention or is there a greater consciousness that determines our existence? And is this simply more philosophy or solely a product of having too much time on my hands?

The point is that I feel closer to understanding something elusive about life because I am less distracted by activities I once was involved in. I feel like my pain is the third rail of the subway line; feeding me the sparks of electricity I need to drive my consciousness into discovering more about my purpose. Not philosophically, but in reality. Ironically, I feel as if my catastrophic event is providing meaning to my life.

Recent events have shown me the positive and negative aspects of my former life and the new process that is unfolding. Why have I been chosen? Am I needed to help others or is this journey really about me being exposed to the clarity of the unshadowed path? The fact I am asking these questions points toward answers or a process that reveals answers. Is the demonstration that I experienced a catastrophe and then consequently began a new life an indication that there are hidden realities, alternate worlds that are already in existence? I long to go deeper and have the answers to these questions revealed. For now, I am at a loss.

Insecurity

There is also a bit of worry for me when my mind begins to wander. Not the kind of creative wandering when the formless is being formed; when the seed of an idea begins to take shape and find direction. There is a joy in the process of that wandering creativity. But, in the floating, disconnected wandering that I am frequently going through, are my feet actually touching the ground?

I remember as a kid how I flung my head back, spread my arms wide and turned and turned in place. How the spinning produced dizziness. How the world was no longer on an even keel. How giddy it made me feel. Now, this confusion of reality is not so much fun. I feel I need the security of the ground.

The events of October 2006 periodically float to the surface of my consciousness and make me wonder...how is it that both my car and my life were thrown far off course by that collision? How is it that I had so little control and could not prevent that from happening? After all, aren't I my own best protector? Was I not a dependable provider for my family?

Unfortunately, even three years later, I have been experiencing a wavering center; a melting core. And this feeling of liquefying and dissolving continues to produce a sense of dis-ease; a loss of knowing that fuels my own sense of inadequacy. But none of this focus or lack of focus is outside my self. So the question becomes where does my self begin and end? Is there any separation between the two? Is there any separation at all? And is the wavering center really a gentle touching upon the super huge, infinite and incomprehensible consciousness of All That Is?

When it comes down to this moment, I can only wonder what part I play in this cosmic theatre and whether my life-changing event is merely highlighting the reality of the myriad roles contained within me.

Rebuilding

Being alive, I hunger for the food of life. I cannot stop, nor do I wish to stop my need to express what is transpiring, to define the walkabout. But within this need, this desire, I have the knowledge that no personal or artistic expression can truly define the vision quest. Does my hunger translate into writing a play? Just as advanced strategy alters the way we play games, so does the desire to "express" drive my life force. Within its nature, the walkabout contains the seed of miraculousness and joy which is expressed through spontaneity. I desperately want that food for my soul, yet my wandering may produce no nourishment, no tangible results at all.

I am so unsteady, so unsure of the next step that it seems as if results appear as a distant dream. My priority is "defining" and clarifying the moment to regain my balance. I feel the game is out of my control; as if I am diving headlong into the rabbit hole with the rush of indistinct objects filling my vision. The blur of the unknown heightens my fear, and like thick glue, its opaque depth masks the clarity of knowing. I feel I will never understand my changes unless I release my preconceived notions into the sea of possibility and discard the old rules of the game. While my bruised body continues to tumble down the rabbit hole, I trust that the protective safety net of understanding will envelop me.

It is terribly unsatisfying being limited to imagining the quality of the result. The deeply satisfying taste of the result is only implied because the process of me achieving this state of being continues to shift. The core, balanced solidity I imagined I needed, or worse, believed existed, was nothing more than a collection of indistinct sands rolling, compacting, and reforming into an infinite arrangement of potentials. It became apparent to me that the creation of life, while mysterious and unfathomable and exemplified by my "new" self, and not the idea of results, was the only choice that mattered. It was life that possessed substance and form.

When I felt I was becoming invisible, both a survival mode and an active purpose became engaged. Like the single bulb illuminating the dank, infrequently visited basement, a possibility of living life in a different way was illuminated. I felt that these new-found rules gave renewed meaning to life. Life was no longer a "thing to do" but rather a magnifying glass that intensified my awareness.

Emerging out of this heightened alertness grew realizations that altered forever how I looked at life and myself in the grand scheme of things. I realized that the awakening of Self into the moment IS the true awareness. I understood that playing the game and being productive is an outward manifestation and that the quality of "being" is an inward realization in which there is no longer an outward/inward difference. I further understood that the structure and rules of society are impersonal and arbitrary but that the heartbeat of life is the elusive "I Am." This realization was huge.

Being "me" is the ultimate expression of consciousness made manifest, the totality of All That Is embodied and reflected in form. My having thoughts, feelings and desires is how consciousness tempers and shapes this ever-changing universe. The "me" is a shout to the universe that I exist. Due to the circumstances of my "event," when my brain shut down random input and memory, the shout of "here I am" became less self centered and transmuted itself into a more uninhibited voice of expression. This voice was my innocent self being elevated to a more vital, hungry and conscious position in the panorama of life. If one imagines a primitive grunt or the scream of the woman whose child has been cruelly killed, one can more deeply understand what the tenor of this "here I am" shout represents. In my ongoing experience, the unfolding of this new self as an expression of a more fundamental truth has become my reason for living.

Role of Memory

How is it possible or even reasonable to assert that the brain shutting down and the loss of memories can further my understanding? It appears contradictory that all the knowledge I learned over a lifetime does not actually further my knowing. Yet, upon closer examination I can gather handfuls of "facts" and summarily discard most of them because they are not facts but either half-truths or the product of statements by limited individuals believing that what they are teaching is gospel.

The jumble of memories is like sectors of a hard drive, so is it fair for me to ask if memories are bad sectors, dead weights, an encumbrance dragging me down? Or is the freedom of being memory-free a gateway into a more unlimited frame? In my specific case, because of my brain injury, a number of events, words, names and sequences have become inaccessible. Since I am not a brain specialist I have no understanding as to whether these forgotten memories are no longer inside the brain or whether they have been wiped out. I believe these memories exist but no longer play an interactive part in my ongoing existence.

When in conversation with people, it is fascinating to observe their reaction when I cannot remember a mutually shared event. There is a look of sadness in their eyes, even pity, that I have become something less than them. My fascination arises from the fact that I see their emotions, withdrawal, judgment and dismissive attitude in such clarity. Prior to my collision I did not feel the depth and texture of someone else in this way. Is this a blessing or curse? Now that parts of my slate have been partially erased there is far more space for these other emotions and experiences to enter. The writing on the chalk board of my brain is fresh and clear. I am excited that the textures have a new set of meanings because they are pristine and not encumbered by past colorations. But the normal, everyday world is balanced on the edge of old and new; past history helping to determine a new course of action.

Without having the resource of certain pages of history, can I function in the world? Can my actions and insights be taken seriously? Will I do something insane because, for example, I don't remember that a lit match can cause the entire house to burn down? While these questions might appear extreme, to the disabled person the world is constantly exerting pressure to conform and be real. Yet in my new-found awareness, the idea of real has less value than the possibility of Being.

Here is another example of how memory assumes a position in recovery. If I had experienced a major stroke and lost huge blocks of memory, then relearning language, speech, movement, etc. would be the activity creating memories. Most of us who have experienced a traumatic event have not been so critically injured as with a major stroke, however, our memory bank has been impacted and changed. For example, the reference points of my world view might have been altered so that what I thought I believed or understood no longer stands as strongly under the scrutiny of my new self. This can be reflected in my new self being fearful of noise or being unable to recognize the danger in crossing the street. Even neuroscientists do not know how the new memory inputs will structure our thoughts, help define our new self, or even how this new self will interact with the world.

I cannot stress enough how much value can be added by allowing these fresh memories to form a healthier self than existed prior to the life-changing event. A self-pitying, woe-is-me attitude can set the foundation for a lifetime of suffering. A more positive "handle what life has presented me" attitude awakened me into a lifetime of creativity and possibility. Pain might be an ongoing component within both attitudes but the manner in which I handled the pain made the difference between managing the world with a degree of joy and satisfaction or falling into negativity and bleakness of spirit. Ultimately, I am the one who gains or loses by the direction taken in terms of attitude.

Resources:

Anatomy of the Spirit by Caroline Myss

Chapter Twenty-Six

FORGIVENESS AND GRATITUDE

"Don Juan assured me that in order to accomplish the feat of making myself miserable I had to work in a most intense fashion, and that it was absurd. I had now realized I could work just the same in making myself complete and strong. 'The trick is in what one emphasizes,' he said. 'We either make ourselves miserable, or we make ourselves strong. The amount of work is the same.'"
- Carlos Castaneda –
Journey to Ixtlan

* * * *

"O admirable necessity! O powerful action! What mind can penetrate your nature? What language can express this marvel?
- Leonardo DaVinci –

I have witnessed the whiners, the martyrs, the deniers, the alarmists, the attackers, the analysts, the I-deserve-this ers, the fighters, the blamers, the sufferers, the lost, the weak, the strong, and so on. There are so many types of individuals that to box in and judge any single one is doing a disservice to the capabilities, motives, and ultimate outcomes that can be seen or imagined. I have seen the weak rising to the occasion, the average Joe giving true understanding to the caregiver, the lost finding purpose, and the desperate and confused finding clarity, calm and comfort in their disease or disability. These are all elements I experienced in the miracle of this process, a process initiated by an event and overcome through attitude.

There are any numbers of scenarios leading up to the life-changing event that may have caused the painful situation we find ourselves in. Someone else might actually have instigated it. They might have been in the middle of road rage and sped up in anger when suddenly their car was out of control and an accident ensued. Or our road rage might have caused a collision that victimized us. In both examples the attitude about the event lays the groundwork for the subsequent healing process.

If we feel guilty about our own rage then we need to forgive ourselves and get on with the business of healing. If we were the victim, then it is equally vital to forgive the person who caused the event because without forgiving them we are ruled by our need to hold onto blame. When we refuse to forgive, we cannot take the responsibility for our healing.

Once catastrophic events have occurred and been moved into the past, the only issue remaining is how we deal with the present. As ugly and painful as it may be, we are the solitary traveler upon that road and it is up to us to handle that reality so that we are living life and not descending into death.

Standing still amidst the rush of humanity, is it any wonder that society determines who my identity is as defined by the reflection of those around me? It seems I have been raised to believe that this mirroring process clarifies who I appear to be. But standing alone after the lights have dimmed, all pretenses fade and there is no longer the fear of my being observed. If I wish, I can choose to project negativity as if I need to pump up my anger in order to overcome a nemesis. Or I can savor the flash of being alive, of my personal humanity, in order to relish in the simple delight of the moment. Now relaxed, the unobstructed sunset on the horizon beckons me to release all separation and breathe in the magnificence of the moment. I realize that no person or outside force can disempower me. It was here where the line between victim and instigator began to disintegrate.

All of us have had the experience of thinking something occurred or was said that made us angry or confused only to find out later that we did not have the complete picture or misunderstood what was actually spoken. By discovering the truth of what happened, as in road rage, we can shift our thought process onto the correct path. Once I have a clearer picture of reality I can choose to release my anger or confusion and then watch it dissipate as if it never existed. What an amazing truth! By shifting perspective I can alter the continuum of my personal reality. This attitude shift is invaluable because it reveals a more harmonious way of being. In my situation this shift opened the possibility for reduced pain and a more hopeful outcome.

When I was victimized by a man driving his truck while he was high on drugs, my life as I knew it changed forever. Naturally, anger and blame arose, with many people being hostile towards the man who hit me. But an interesting progression of emotions and memories was directing me through my days, and these emotions had little to do with the driver of the truck that hit me. If you have ever had a traumatic event, you probably recollect what you were feeling in its wake and I am certain your experience was similar to mine. The focus for me was not my job, the bills that needed to be paid, the calls I wanted to return or the theatre tickets I had with my wife. Nor was my focus on the person who almost killed me. Something quite unexpected was transpiring. I found myself wondering where I was, what caused the terrible pain I was experiencing, and even more importantly, how thankful I felt to both be alive and be able to see my wife and children again. The degree of joy, even through the pain-killing drug haze, was so all encompassing that the idea of blame was not even a consideration. This is the power of love and the uplifting feeling of familial ecstasy.

Over time, I became aware that the root of my strangely positive feeling was attitude. By looking at myself through the lens of thankfulness, I was eliminating the negativity of anger and blame. In this process, I found I was free from feeling angry at another person for hurting me. Instead, I was able to take the energy of anger, blame, hopelessness and fear and direct it towards the real feelings that had sustainability: the love of my family and the gratitude of still being alive.

Both these sets of feelings are powerful, and each would propel me along divergent paths. When I chose the positive path instead of the negative, I immediately embarked on healing. By taking attitude into account in the healing process, my redefinition of self became an integral part of my healing.

My life-changing event took place in less than two seconds but I was ill prepared for the impact it would have on who I would become for the rest of my life. No one had taught me how to disidentify from who I had been my entire life. Consequently, I did not know how to establish the space in which to reinvent myself.

The imaginary walls of identification felt like the boundaries of a house cat, which, living outside has, by its nature, imposed a hundred yard radius of existence to remain within the safety of home. To the cat, when peering across the lawn, the trees beyond are but distant possibilities, frightening in their vast unknown quality. Like the cat, I too had constructed a safe environment from which to function.

Within our safe world we identify with and participate in many different activities which we take for granted. Were you an avid bicycle rider who can no longer ride? Did you rock climb but can now no longer use one of your arms? Did you dance on a regular basis but can now no longer use one leg for more than a few minutes? Since we are examining a life-altering event and not the advances of old age, this ceasing of regular, pleasurable, even professional activities happening in the blink of an eye is traumatic.

Is it logical or even intelligent to assume that the transition from the old into the new would snap into place immediately and without problems? Of course not! I discovered that it is our attitude toward these life changes that is most critical. We must allow our attitude to assist us in this most difficult transition. Relearning words I lost because of brain trauma was understandably frustrating, however, with an attitude of expectancy about this new learning and welcoming incremental change, the reacquisition of speaking skills became a joyous experience. This is the gift of attitude.

How often has it occurred that when you thought positive thoughts about someone that they suddenly called you out of the blue? Or when you kept repeating what a stupid car you had, the next thing you knew the car would not start; or worse, your anger ended up in a fender bender? Are these causes and effects connected? Did your thoughts create the subsequent action? An entire field of psycho-spirituality directly addresses this question. They posit that when you think something with strength and clarity, the event has now occurred in the unmanifested world and it is only a matter of time before it occurs in the manifested world. This is not to say that a negative action is inevitable or irreversible, but, by altering ones thoughts into a more positive, less angry framework, an alternative result can occur. This is the aspect of attitude I am addressing.

When we are looking at and living in the midst of pain and despair, it is a remote concept that we can change our reality by changing our attitude. Nonetheless, it is precisely this attitude that needs addressing. During my third time on the operating table I was aware enough to give the nurses a few "affirmations" to be said out loud during my operation. It is a recognized fact that patients under anesthesia or even in a comatose state continue to hear what is being said to them. For this reason, only positive statements should be spoken by anyone in the Operating Room while you are under the surgeon's knife. In addition, I was able to give the nurses a CD of music to be played while I was in the OR. This was my favorite play list and the idea was that it would nourish my subconscious while I was under anesthesia on the operating table. Both the affirmations and music were positive attitude strokes; ways in which my body could perceive itself healed before my mind could post roadblocks to my wellness.

Pain and despair can overwhelm even the strongest patients. By carefully planting and nourishing positive thoughts, another path can be chosen. By taking this fresh road we can walk on firmer ground, find a more secure balance and perceive light instead of the prevailing darkness that appears to suffocate our progress. This is not to say that we cannot heal without a positive attitude. After all, the energy of anger, of wanting to get stronger while feeling weak, can fuel our recovery. The power of anger, directed toward health and recovery is a slice of focused attitude. But by broadening the scope of positive attitude adjustments, we can feel more hopeful. This, in turn, aids in approaching the process of recovery in ways that enable us to grow, change and become more whole as human beings.

For most of us in the wake of a traumatic event, full recovery does not exist. But the prospect of partial recovery in a full new self is awe inspiring and quite miraculous. Toward this end, a "woe is me" attitude is detrimental to full or partial recovery. By being mired in a woe is me attitude, we negate the opportunity of realizing the new self. Wearing the coat of positivity magnetizes a wealth of possible positive outcomes to us. If, by thinking strongly of someone creates them calling you, just imagine what thinking strongly about your wellness will create!

What is this "new" you? What level of recovery will you achieve? These answers are unknown, however, like the excitement of opening up a birthday present, when the ribbons and wrapping paper are cast aside and the box is opened, this new me was a gift from the great creative Spirit. This unmanifested Source energy was the clay to be shaped by my positivity. When I maintained an attitude of wonder and miraculousness, I was able to be joyful and applaud the small but significant changes I made during recovery. My re-formed self was different, surprising, and indeed new, and by welcoming him in I was able to cut off negativity at the knees and stand tall with my positive outlook.

Emergence of Hope

In viewing the world it is obvious there are vast numbers of people damaged in one way or another. For me, it was just as important to allow my emotions to empathize with others as it was to focus and generate strength for my own journey. I had never experienced such personal destruction before, so this journey was new and frightening. Seeking the help of a wide range of professionals who were trained in the way of recovery was equally as valid as plugging away daily and doing the suggested exercises by myself. Setting my mind, my heart and my will upon a road littered with setbacks and seemingly insurmountable hurdles was instrumental in me taking the first baby steps toward recovery.

Once I embarked on this trip to a still undetermined end, another door slowly squeaked open. Faint and indistinct, this door revealed a glimmer of light off in the distance. The path of this light was Hope. Not the kind of hope one hopes when it is late, that the store is still open, but the kind of hope that infuses oneself with a possibility that something, recovery in my case, actually exists.

I felt that I had to trust in something as elusive as hope. I knew what it felt like to want something; to hope and pray that a goal will be achieved. But when the bottom line basic functioning of my body is the issue, hope of success takes on enormous value with an entirely new meaning. While I was hopeful, I was also so fearful of failure that it took all my effort to remain focused on the positive.

The picture of my recovery was incomplete because no one, from surgeon to therapist and family members knew what the final outcome was going to be. What would I be capable of doing? How would my brain function? Would I ever be a self sufficient person again? In the beginning, words of encouragement were spoken often and passionately. It was vital to believe in myself and reinforce the positive emotional support given to me so I could take action. A major aspect in initially taking steps toward recovery was having the belief that my life was not over and that I had the power to define what my life was to become by being proactive in the healing process. Given the idea that I did not know what my "new" self was going to look like, I was free to compose it like a musician finding the correct notes in a symphony. Growing through my own process of trial and error, I could then observe and help others in their quest. No longer encumbered by needing to judge others' progress I was able to reach out beyond my injured self and embrace the desire and growth of others in their varying catastrophic conditions.

By observing other damaged people I was able to assume a clearer perspective of the extent of my damage. In addition, with the knowledge that each of us is at a different developmental point, it became evident that by encouraging others I was further validating my own work. By taking the time to listen to others in worse shape than I, I was actually making it easier to listen to myself. What began as a solitary catastrophe evolved into a more humanistic outlook and sensitivity towards others and myself. I realized that this outlook is controlled by the mind and its expression is attitude.

Resources:

The Power of Positive Thinking by Norman Vincent Peale
The Tibetan Art of Positive Thinking: Skillful Thought for Successful Living by Christopher Hansard
Positive Affirmations: 92 Affirmations That Apply Positive Quotes And Positive Words To Banish Negative Thinking by Gary Vurnum

Chapter Twenty-Seven

WORKING WITH PAIN

"We say that we cannot bear our troubles but when we get to them we bear them."
- Ning Lao T'ai-t'ai –

"God gives food to every bird, but does not throw it into the nest."
- Monteganrin proverb -

When I was five years old I had a horribly painful accident. I was rushed to the hospital to await reconstructive surgery on my left elbow the following morning. The key experience, however, was during the night prior to surgery. Although my arm was immobilized and I was sedated, I moved my body and arm slightly on the hospital bed. When I did, the level of pain was more than a five year old could tolerate.

During those moments of agony an incredible and miraculous thing occurred. My inner self spontaneously separated from my body. It seemed to do that in order to relieve me of pain. What happened was the self that was in my body, aligned with emotions and thoughts became disconnected from that alignment and in disconnecting I no longer felt pain and no longer had a feeling about my current situation. I had a direct experience of being separated from my body while still being alive. I experienced myself floating upward like a helium balloon until I stopped, resting on the ceiling. From that vantage point, feeling perfectly intact, I looked down upon my prostrate body and I saw the temporary splint on my elbow, the room I was in, and the nurse entering and exiting through the door into the well lit hallway.

I did not have any form of magical insight into what was happening; I could not read the mind of the nurse or suddenly know everything that was about to occur in the future. The only truth was that I was able to be separate from my body and still maintain the living, breathing nature of my body. In this way I was able to be free from pain because I was not residing in my body where the pain could be felt. This separation did not feel odd or unusual. Since I was only five years old and my intellect was not yet developed, I did not have a pre-judgment to negate this truth, no matter how strange it appeared. After all, I was existing in two places at the same time!

Later in life I learned that the word astral projection defines the state I was in. Though unproven by Western science, the idea and experience of the Soul separating from the body is mentioned in Ecclesiastes, is referred to in Theosophy, is part of ancient Egyptian practices and is foundational in Taoism and Hinduism. With practice, this state can be entered into at will. Furthermore, the astral body is not limited by the ceiling of a room but can be extended into the far reaches of the universe. The only descriptive similarity is like having a waking dream or a totally lucid sleeping dream in which all the details are remembered. In an advanced developmental state, the actions in the dream can be controlled. In the pain-ridden state, the feeling of pain can also be controlled. I cannot inhabit this separated state at all times, but experiencing it just once has given me insight into the nature of pain and the potential for controlling it.

Having the belief you can control or master some degree of outcome, in this case pain, is an integral part of actually being able to achieve it. This belief is an attitude; the difference between descending into pain and the relief in rising above it. When Helen Keller narrates that her deafness and blindness is not a limitation but an opportunity to expand into the awareness and creativity of the universe, the opportunity she is describing is what I am labeling "attitude."

We have heard many adages that state "you are what you eat" or "think positive thoughts" or "project success and you will achieve it." These aphorisms wash over us every day. We have been inundated so often by New Age concepts, self help and "how to" books, that we have become numb to the truth they are trying to express. In fact, we often turn off to the message and negate the power of this reality. But this truth is not glib or shallow or a parlor trick. No charlatan need convince us that this attitude adjustment works; each of us has had first-hand experience to validate its success.

When this attitude adjustment is employed in the transmuting of pain, it not only demonstrates what is real but what is possible. This tweaking of attitude has within it the actual power of practicality resulting in diminished pain as well as the potential power of unlimited consciousness resulting in a change in the state of being through focused thought. This is an enormous lesson that becomes applicable in a wealth of areas. For my purposes, the lessening of physical suffering was reason enough to apply this understanding.

I became aware that whatever attitude I held in regard to my pain literally made the pain stronger or weaker, overwhelming or manageable. Once I understood that both possibilities were woven into my attitude, I faced a choice. I observed how many damaged people allow their pain to grow, expect others to do the work for them, rely on medications to make them feel better, and even desire for the pain to continue so that others will pay attention to them. Other people chose to see the arc of pain as a natural progression of mild to intense and back to mild again. These people inserted themselves consciously into the flow of pain and thereby managed it more effectively. My choice was to model this and learn pain management.

I became aware that I could give shape to the pain and its movement from mild to severe, and then deconstruct the overall picture into its components. These individual elements comprising pain, once observed, become, in a strange way separated from suffering. When I was able to place the location of the pain and rate its degree of intensity, essentially not taking the pain personally, I became more objective in what I needed to assist me in relieving and managing it. By adjusting my attitude towards my experience, I was able to work more effectively with my pain, anxiety and fear. By shifting attitude, I was no longer embroiled in anger as well as pain. I now stood at the center of the storm raging around me with the knowledge that I could maintain some semblance of equilibrium in the midst of the maelstrom. The tools necessary to handle this storm needed to be learned but the key to opening the toolbox was my attitude. For me, attitude was not simply an intellectual understanding. Like scraping away the rust of past beliefs, my attitude needed to be revealed and activated through my choices.

Since pain is inside me, I fantasized that my elusive desire to be whole would blanket my pain. But this magical thinking masks reality. How does the leverage of desire to be pain free act in conjunction with an IV tube dripping attitude into my bloodstream? The truth is that the IV drip is nothing more than the beating reminder of inevitability. The medicine dissolved within the liquid a symbolic catalyst for change. The button I push to administer the dose, an existential reminder of failure and hope. These opposing emotions, inseparable from the engine of attitude, are the rays of brightness that produce clarity.

I need to observe this clarity as if I was a mythic God, apart, aloof and impersonal. I have to embrace the need for clarity as I would envelop a newborn in my protective resilience. Most importantly, it is crucial that I love the clarity with a fatalistic exuberance, knowing this moment could be my last. Rock. Paper. Scissors. The only winning strategy is attitude.

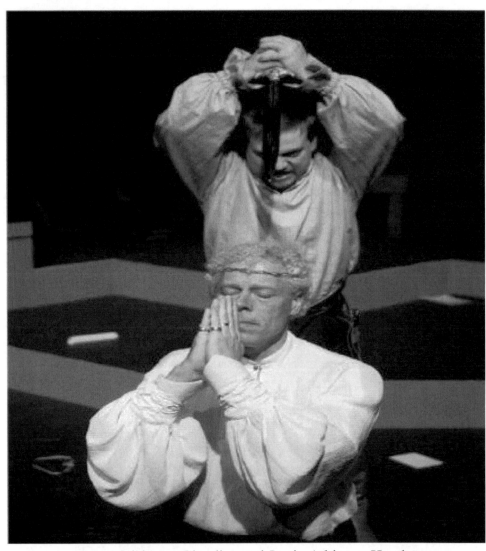

Marc Maislen as Claudius and Justin Atkins as Hamlet
Photo: ChrisGraamansPhotography.com

Chapter Twenty-Eight

A NEW TRUTH

"The curious paradox is that when I accept myself just as I am, then I can change."
- Carl Rogers –

"Once we truly know that life is difficult – once we truly understand and accept it – then life is no longer difficult. Because once it is accepted, the fact that life is difficult no longer matters."
- M. Scott Peck –
The Road Less Traveled

A New Reality

I remember gently slumbering in the deep grass of summer; the buoyancy of the grass duplicating the weightless support of the salty ocean. As I awaken, inching toward consciousness, my eyes adjust to the still plane of the lake. Not yet aware that my head is angled downward, it appears that I am gazing at the blue sky and puffy white clouds. I am immersed in this sight with innocent wonder as my heart flutters with joy. With a start I fully awaken into reality, aware that it is the reflection of the sky that is etched with clarity on the lake's motionless surface. It is not the sky itself that was touching my heart but its reflection.

Ancient mariners had detailed maps of the ocean in order to avoid rocks and eddies that could shipwreck them and spell disaster. My "event" thrust me into a universe with far fewer maps and guideposts than I had previously relied upon. For example, to navigate the world I had to learn to correctly work the controls of an automobile. But there is no template when using an automobile (to get from one place to another) for enjoying the car's motion, remaining calm in the face of traffic jams, and feeling the miracle of the engine itself. The actual mechanics of driving is a minor memory when viewed in the context of the expanded consciousness of driving. The ancient mariners, similar to the modern extreme sports enthusiasts, lived on this sensory edge. One aspect of themselves was devoted to the adventure, risk and freedom of their quest while another was simultaneously maintaining a margin of safety that would enable them to survive and experience the rush of exploring uncharted territory.

After a traumatic event, the world can appear as precariously balanced as being on the edge of a chasm, as feeling the frightening pull of a tornado, as being bombarded by the deafening sound of an explosion or the overwhelming power of Niagara Falls. It was critical that I address my differences, my lack of memory, and the ever changing face of the world, in a manner that would not sever my new-found connection to the universe. I approached this as a student; voraciously learning all my brain could handle.

A New Self

The exploration of the unknown has traditionally been the province of the risk taker, the artist, the entrepreneur, the great teacher. To achieve my wholeness I had to adopt more of those qualities. By surrounding myself with others on a similar mission and finding the fearless people around me, I was helped immeasurably with my emergence into the current world. The abyss is no less deep nor is the tumult any smoother to maneuver through, but the experience of it, my part in the totality, has grown far beyond my old self. I can now smile kindly upon others who are judging my limp because I have the knowledge that I am happy for them in their ability to walk unencumbered.

The importance of validating and upholding my "new self" was probably the most important commitment I had ever made. It was already my experience that people feel sorry for you after a life-altering event. A wheelchair, scars, and dismemberment are all external appearances that cause fear, revulsion, pity and uninformed accusations in others. So my strength in staying the course of discovering my new self was the hardest, most concentrated action I had ever taken. This could be compared to a toddler learning how to walk and talk. Isn't it interesting how cute we think infants are in their struggle to become and integrate in the world? Then why do adults think less of those of us who have survived a life-altering event when we are struggling to become our new selves? Their fear and insecurity in relating to us as "damaged goods" should not deter us from our mission to be whole; to add to the harmony and growth of the world. But this learning curve is very steep and not easy to traverse.

The uncharted territory of my new self embodies the thrill of skydiving, the restlessness of awaiting the results of an exam and the tentativeness of asking a person out on a date. It is no easy task to maintain the balance between these energetic states of being while still pursuing a course of healing. When I was finally able to look at myself in the mirror, see the numerous scars lacing my body and not get thrown back into a warmer and fuzzier memory of myself, this flash of realization was the turning point which enabled me to take on the difficulties of the course ahead.

The new self is both real and metaphorical. The symbol of this new self is the mirror. I remember my shock when I first looked in the mirror and saw a different person. Was it the scars that now marked my body? Or was it the tubes that were coming out of my body? Or is my twisted smile really a sarcastic grimace of some unknown person on the other side of the glass?

Before the metaphorical self is addressed, the real self requires quite a lot of time in order to incorporate itself into everyday living. I needed a walker to get from one place to another and at times I could only shuffle my feet in order to walk. What about my not having the strength to open a bottle; or that my fingers no longer open and close easily or with fine muscular control? And how about my lacking flexibility to raise my arm above my shoulder?

No longer thinking I'm in a dream, I know I need help getting dressed. I am ready to go out, or at least want to be dressed for getting around the house. I breathe in and exhale a sense of satisfaction. I look at myself and wonder how it is that I cannot dress myself. I am no longer saddened by this. I breathe in a sense of accomplishment. I smile and laugh quietly at the absurdity that I cannot dress myself. I breathe and nod at the understanding that I am different but okay. I breathe and look at myself again. My new self is dressed and ready for action.

This new self is me. It is not my wife's or children's or therapist's or my doctor's. I own this new self like a custom made suit that fits only me. This new self might demand the attention of others or ask for help from people around me, but it does so without the distractions of work, housekeeping, and other things. I am spending more time than is comfortable being with myself. I must remember my self is just starting out again. This is a new beginning. Whether I am afraid to wrinkle my new suit or get it dirty, this is my suit to wear, break in, and be proud of when I face the world.

In the past, how many times had I said to myself, "If I were 18 again…." or "If I could start again I would try something different." In a sick cosmic twist, I have been given the opportunity to fulfill these thoughts. The fantasy of dream fulfillment is open to me. I have been given the privilege of acting this out. I have suffered irreversible trauma as a metaphor for change and breaking the mold. The relevant issue is how I embrace the challenge of starting this new dream life.

I ask myself, "Why would an intelligent human being choose suffering and pain as a vehicle for change?" If I examine the other ridiculously stupid choices I've made, such as jobs that I detested; relationships that did not work; clothes and styles that were unflattering; and many, many more, the picture is clear. The indistinct edges of my former day to day existence barely touched upon suffering and pain, but by bringing the lens of pain and suffering into sharper focus I simply made this choice more dramatic. If the truth be told, I probably needed this level of extreme drama in order to get me to act upon "something else""

The price I am paying for this rare opportunity is to no longer have the same physical and/or mental skills I once possessed. Therefore, certain life options cannot be explored, like continuing to be a dancer. It is important for me to understand that although this and other possibilities have to be dismissed, additional options will now present themselves. My new self needs to be willing to explore these hidden, as yet undiscovered places within me that hold the keys to fulfillment in my "new" future. Without this inquisitive opening of my eyes I will remain in a state of denial.

By exploring my adult life through dance, American Mime and theatre I acquired the tools to lead a creative life. What I learned was how to look at myself and situations fearlessly so that the center, the creativity of possibilities could be revealed. My touchstone was always expression through movement. By accepting my diminished ability to move my body in the "old" manner, I in no way weakened the creativity, accomplishment and gratification produced by giving 100% to the "new" me.

When I feel sorry for myself that I no longer have the skills to be on stage again I only have to remind myself that a lifetime of knowledge about my stage technique can be taught to others. I might not be able to continue as a professional dancer but I can work with disabled children or young adults so they might express themselves and find fulfillment through dance and theatre. Embracing the act of teaching again is helping me lead a productive, post-collision, fulfilling life. What an unusual, meaningful and unexpected gift!

Chapter Twenty-Nine

THE NEW SELF

Recollection from the Hospital Bed:

"In my dream I am running away from some shapeless, unknown threat. I peel off my face believing I will no longer be recognized. The environment gets hotter burning my new face. I peel this new face off. When I look up, a huge metal and glass building appears in front of me reflecting my image. Just as I get close enough to see my face I wake up."

* * * *

"If you wanna make the world a better place,
Take a look at yourself and then make a change."
"Man in the Mirror"
- Ballard & Garrett sung by Michael Jackson -

* * * *

"We have often heard it said that God never closes one door unless he opens another. It is a great comfort to know we never really lose when we believe, for any defeat can be turned to good if we will absorb the lesson in it."
- Joyce Hifler -

Once the life-altering event has occurred, there is no going back, no reverse gear, no instant replay. It is like attending the funeral of a dear friend and knowing you will never see them again except in the realm of memory. This is the same for us. The old self is dead. Long live the "new self!"

In fact, while other people continue to address you by your name, underneath the surface they, too, are looking at you as someone new.

166

We have established the pattern and tenor of our lives through years of repetition, habit, likes and dislikes, and the general ebb and flow of existence. Suddenly, this image, while appearing on the surface as the same image previously understood, no longer contains the same content. If you can imagine a predominately blue colored painting suddenly photo-shopped into a red painting, you can recognize how the painting changes in meaning.

Our inner Self does not reconstruct itself because of the external scars life impresses upon us. We might no longer have a hand, become blind, have a stroke, or even be in survival mode due to war or famine. Outwardly, we might make the adjustment to having only one hand or be driven by our need for food to survive, but internally we remain the same. We are, in spite of everything, still ourselves. These external scars or disabilities, however, are viewed by others and in turn they form an impression upon the beholder as to who we are. It is not uncommon as we age to experience looking in the mirror and seeing an older version of our self, remark how we still think and feel like a twenty year old. Someone meeting you for the first time has no idea of your past abilities and therefore looks and judges you in your present state.

I can hold up a mirror to scrutinize myself; even discredit what I see. But when I go beyond this personal objectification, I can only ask, who am I, really?

The clock representing our time on Earth ticks downward, edging ever closer to the finality of zero. When times runs out, life's tumultuous course can be viewed as a danger zone leading to the specter of abandoned dreams left in the portfolio of youth. So what remains? Is a pristine new truth revealed in frenzy, like the frantic unwrapping of a present? Or does the revelation of Self unfold in the almost imperceptible nodding of "ah ha" moments? Hopefully, the layering of a lifetime of cynicism is not so deeply ingrained that the magic and illumination of wonder is incorrectly dismissed as illusion. We must fight to stay awake and aware.

We know that the substance in the mirror's reflection is indistinct, at best. Just as the dimly lit dining room washes over us with the illusion of softness, youth and self importance, the modern fluorescents accentuate the cold, hard and pallid quality of our skin. Is either of these reflections valuable in assessing who we are?

Wake up to the idea that the new self is not just new to outsiders. The deeper and more vital understanding is that the new self is new to us, too. When I awoke after the collision, the world was no longer what I once knew it to be. And while it was obvious that others viewed me in a different way, the more difficult task was being able to view myself as being different. Whereas growing older, yet still feeling like a twenty year old is taken in stride as a natural experience of self through the stages of aging, the surprise of suddenly awakening into a less able self is not natural at all.

If I can look at my new self as a person re-born, I am on the healthy path. Since I am not invoking religion, what does this rebirth entail? To begin, embracing the idea of my self as a new person is so disconnected from my normal reality that it borders on the impossible; yet, this concept must be adopted, assimilated and acted upon. When I thought of my old self as a physically dominating person, biking and climbing, running from place to place, and teaching others dance, mime and personal strength training, I was comfortable in this state of being. But confronting my lack or diminished ability in these areas, I was thrust into sadness, depression and a whirl of confusion as to what my life would be like as I progressed into the future. How was I supposed to function without the skills and ways of interacting that I was accustomed to? Could I lead a productive life? Would I be able to be happy as I moved into the future?

The key to answering these questions resided in both my attitude and my willingness to actually be re-born. When I was originally born leaving my mother's womb and bursting into this life, the transition was natural. My current rebirth into my new self, however, was fraught with heavy baggage. This rebirth needed to be dealt with physically, intellectually, emotionally and spiritually. Clearly this transition was not going to be easy. But all things considered, there was no time to delay or deny this rebirth if I truly wanted to claim, as me, the new person I was becoming.

I only needed to observe the world to see how "Mother Earth" is continually providing an ongoing model of rebirth. It's like when I find myself in the back yard after a huge rain storm. I look down and see my bare feet and toes squishing into the soft, muddy ground. I cannot remember the last time I stood outside without my shoes on. It is as if I am recharging myself from the Source, the Earth.

Looking at a new birth one expects pain and disorientation. After all, the entire landscape is new. But for a newborn, all the energy of parents and family are focused on taking care of them. There is little awareness of what the infant is going through. Most projections about the newborn are about his or her learning what is happening in the real world. Apart from walking, talking and eating, no attention is paid to their perspective of the world. We consider them a blank slate without judgment or perception about what they are seeing and hearing.

My rebirth was quite different. In my current life-altering situation, my new self not only looked at others differently but now had a new past history to reflect upon and use as a reference point. It was not only about how other people were relating to me. It was also about how I was relating to other people. What they did not realize was that I was shocked by my confusion about who THEY were. Sometimes people who appeared in the past to be compassionate were now revealed as manipulators. Even friends that usually came across as funny were now experienced by me as acidic and cutting in their words. Actions once viewed by me as positive and building were revealed as self serving and greedy. Talk about a wakeup call! Just when I considered kicking back and having others help me, the realization that many friends and family members were unrecognizable to me was frightening. I did not want their imprint upon my new self.

This is not to say that everything in the world suddenly became bizarre and incomprehensible. The truth is that life is awash in shades of gray, and as my eyes readjusted to the colors and gradations of the world, so did my emotions adjust to what holds value in this new panorama. My old self might have been thrilled to pass a car on the highway and get to my destination one minute earlier than expected. Now, my new self has no interest in arriving early because my thrill is in enjoying the ride no matter what the traffic pattern reveals. In fact, being calm instead of being enraged has enormous importance to my new self.

Knowing I could not control what others were thinking and feeling about me was a significant hurdle I overcame in the process of accepting who I had become. When letting go of control was coupled with experiencing people in terms of what they were actually doing, I was then able to allow myself to see others as who they are. Unfortunately, this was often an unpleasant surprise for me, although experiencing this newness was a valuable lesson in redefining my new self. I often thought that others were judging me in my disabled state but I realized that a far more important issue was how I was perceiving the outside world. Understanding my own thoughts and feelings were the keys in determining my interaction with the world.

When facing the unknown, the line between ability and inability and clarity versus grayness can be monumentally frustrating. Though a particular action was previously known, like going to the supermarket, this simple action can become an uncomfortable trial. When I went shopping in the past, I proceeded down the aisles and selected items my family needed. My new self cannot remember what we need or can be so intrigued by a colorful jar that I toss it into the cart. Knowing that I need a list and preparing for the visit to the supermarket is difficult. What is important for me to realize is that by defusing frustration through adequate preparation I can prevent anxious moments from becoming overwhelming.

My new self must be given the proper respect and enough time to reorient itself to this new world. Where I once taught others how to improve their athleticism, I now need to discover the key to how my physical changes can first educate myself and then educate others who are facing disabling injuries. If my despair is overwhelming, I have to transmute that negativity into a joy at being alive. When my thoughts and feelings appear inconsequential in the face of physical challenges, it is vital for me to discover how small, incremental changes can be emotionally uplifting.

In the same way as a baby builds feelings and locates what feels pleasurable, I too have to focus on what I am experiencing now. The likes and dislikes of the past no longer have the same credence because my new self is redefining the way in which I experience the world. In the past, when I would multi-task, my attention was split. For example, by spreading butter in the pan while simultaneously beating eggs in the bowl I saved time in making breakfast. But now I need to whisk the eggs and then progress to buttering the pan since multi-tasking is difficult. The upside is that because I am now more aware of each individual activity, I can pay fuller attention to it, and ultimately experience each action more completely. I find I am being rewarded with a deeper satisfaction from the actions I take because I am more fully in the moment.

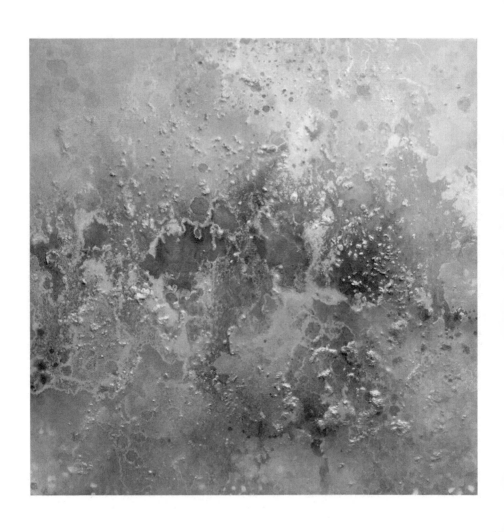

"Vapul 2" by Deborah Barlow, SlowMuse.com

Chapter Thirty

CONNECTED

My recollection on this New Perspective:

"I awaken in the middle of the night. My ears are ringing because my nightmare found me trapped in my car with the Jaws of Life cutting me out. The noise is deafening. I can't stop the noise."

* * * *

"Inside yourself or outside, you never have to change what you see, only the way you see it."
                    - Thaddeus Golas -

I know my experience is personal yet able to be shared with others. I know I am not alone but I can still find myself terribly isolated from the world. I know I have ears and eyes but how I listen and see is vital to being more fully who I am. I know my body will function and survive even when my brain is unconscious and not in control.

Coming full circle out of the dream into reality I breathe in the warmth of the Sun. My body, relaxed and unhurried fills itself with the peace of knowing I am alive and vibrant. I breathe even more deeply. I exhale and smile. I am indeed recovering.

When I now experience my family and friends and interact with people in everyday life, I am not struck by how successful they have become, the quality and cut of their clothes, or their travels and exploits. I am moved by their care, their attention to smaller activities, and how willing they are to be open and vulnerable. Since my collision I have been less interested in how I appear to others, having exchanged that for

how I can participate in being who I am and enabling others to be more themselves.

I understand I will probably never be pain free but that my pain is tempered by the degree of new ability I have achieved. I also understand on a more fundamental level that comparing myself to how I once moved through life is a waste of time. I will never be that man again. By acknowledging and experiencing the joy of who I am now, life has a transcendent quality and a dramatic upside. In my journey through trauma towards recovery I hit rock bottom, but because of the choices I made I now know I do not have to remain there forever. This is a way of living and being that balances the daily pain I still experience with the gift of being alive.

So many people have contributed to my well being. I only pray that I can give back even a fraction of what has been given to me. When my attitude shifted and I committed to wanting to be alive, the world of possibility opened before me. It was eye-opening to experience the wealth of people willing to give of themselves in helpful services to me and others like me. I never knew how vast the network of care givers, therapists and professionals was and how tirelessly they serve people like me day in and day out, devoting themselves to incorporating medicine, science and healing arts with the sole purpose of making our lives happier, healthier and more manageable. This was certainly the case with me.

All our stories are different. The road to recovery is personal. Pain is experienced subjectively and alone. Yet, through the maze of upheaval, my sense of humanity, both for the individual and the collective grew in magnitude transcending my personal belief system and becoming a way for me to embrace others. Pain and need are the common denominators. The desire to live and be integrated into the world has become my underlying driving force. My recovery is no longer reliant upon focusing on pain and loss; it has expanded into a quest for freedom.

All of us are tested throughout our lives. Whether we have the courage to face the challenges and embrace what life offers, is our choice. The test of recovery with its commensurate pain is a difficult path to traverse. But when our attitude, focus, positivity, creativity and will are applied to such a formidable challenge, the resultant gifts of understanding, compassion, self-love and success, while not easily measured, cannot be denied.

Life now has a new complexion for me. The nuances I have experienced and the subtleties I have become aware of continue to feed into my feeling of gratefulness. There is so much to be thankful for; so much love to be shared. It remains a mystery as to why pain and recovery were the gateways for me to experience the miraculousness of life. I do know it was crucial for me to find the strength to pass through these doors and truly experience living.

May you find your inner strength to transcend the challenges on your own unique journey. Good luck on your quest.

APRIL 2012

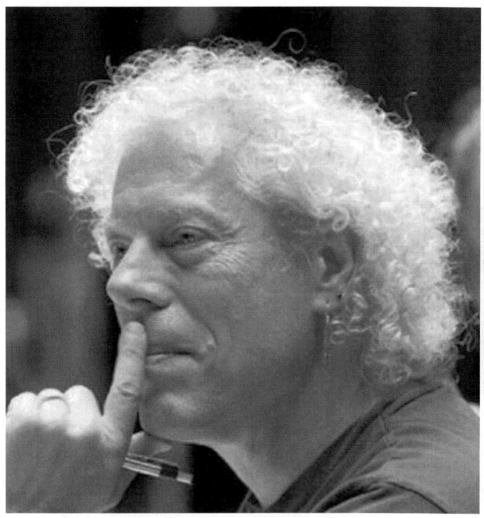

Watching Actors Rehearse while Directing "Speed-the-Plow"
Photo: ChrisGraamansPhotography.com

EPILOGUE

It was a full four and a half years since October 2006, the Spring of 2011, before I was able to participate in what I loved most: theatre. By moving to the Oregon Coast, the pressure of acting or directing on a major stage was removed. The community embraced me as I now was and subsequently the energy given to me uplifted my spirits and enabled me to take the opportunity to again become involved in the Arts. Although I could not participate in musical theatre involving dancing I was able to carve a niche in speaking theatre.

My right arm continues to be a work in progress; moving it fully being quite a challenge. And as long as I do not need to walk non-stop, my hip functions well enough to limit limping. The fact that I am sufficiently recovered to ply my craft at a professional level again empowers me on a daily basis. Memorizing lines, on the other hand, is absurdly challenging. I probably need five times the number of hours other actors need in order to keep the words ordered and available to speak. Nonetheless, I am meeting these challenges with clarity; understanding what it takes to be successful and doing it.

Although I am incapable of playing tennis, I have taken up the piano. The fingers of my right hand are not as fluid as my left but through repetition and stretch they, too, are participating in an activity that I was incapable of approaching two years ago.

My workouts remain a staple of my weekly schedule. I am stronger, more flexible and am finally able to do circuit training. What is truly heartening is I can do half my bike rides on a Spin bike and the other half on the recumbent bike. My hip can withstand the pressure! I am projecting that within the next year I will be capable of road biking. Mountain biking is still an impossibly distant dream.

My wife and I continue to change, grow and thrive. She, too, is participating in theatre; directing and acting. Our involvement in the Arts has reestablished a base of understanding and depth in our relationship that was put on hold. This, in addition to my ability to share in the daily challenges, chores, vacations and appreciation of nature and life makes our marriage one of renewed love and anticipation of what the future has in store.

I drive a car without being frightened, hear a range of sound that does not throw me into an anxiety attack and experience myself as I am, without falling into the web of depression.

My work is not yet complete and I look upon each day as a miracle; a gift of time bestowed on me. In the same way I was snatched from the jaws of death I approach each day with the knowledge that life is so fragile that I dare not disregard its beauty.

Shattered

RESOURCE LIST

OVERVIEW

Fearless: Creating the Courage to Change the Things You Can by Steve Chandler

The Power of Breathing (Self-help and Spiritual series) by Dr. Sukhraj S. Dhillo

A Book of Stress Relief Tips by Kathy Berman

Maps to Ecstasy: The Healing Power of Movement by Gabrielle Roth, John Loudon and Angeles Arrien

It's Your Choice! Decisions That Will Change Your Life by Marjorie McKinnon

The Art of Finding Yourself, At Any Age by Karen Sala

PAIN EXPERIENCE

Dissolving Pain by Les Fehmi and Jim Robbins

The Chronic Pain Management Sourcebook (Lowell House) by David E. Drum

WHY?

To Begin Again by Rabbi Naomi Levy

When Bad Things Happen to Good People by Rabbi Harold Kushner

How to go on Living When Someone You Love Dies by Therese Rando

Tear Soup by Pat Schweibert

The Tibetan Book of Living and Dying: The Spiritual Classic & International Bestseller by Patrick Gaffney

On Death and Dying by Elisabeth Kubler-Ross

THE TRAUMATIZED MARRIAGE

Family Manual, A manual for families of persons with pain by Penney Cowan

CARE GIVING UP CLOSE

The Fearless Caregiver: How to Get the Best Care for Your Loved One and Still Have a Life of Your Own (Capital Cares) by Gary Barg
God Knows Caregiving Can Pull You Apart: 12 Ways to Keep it All Together by Gretchen Thompson
Caregiving: The Spiritual Journey of Love, Loss, and Renewal by Beth Witrogen McLeod

COMPANIONSHIP

Working Like Dogs: The Service Dog Guidebook by Marcie Davis

EXPECTATION

Coping With Family Expectations by Margaret Hill

MEDICATION AND WITHDRAWAL

The Pain Relief Handbook : Self-Help Methods for Managing Pain by Chris Wells, Graham Nown, Chrissie Wells, Ronald Melzack
Overcoming Chronic Pain: A Self-Help Guide Using Cognitive Behavioral Techniques by Frances Cole, Hazel Howden-Leach, Helen Macdonald, Catherine Carus
How to Get Off Psychoactive Drugs Safely: There is Hope. There is a Solution by James Harper N.C. (Author), Jayson Austin N.C. (Contributor)

WHAT IS PROGRESS?

The Tibetan Art of Positive Thinking: Skillful Thought for Successful Living by Christopher Hansard
Positive Affirmations: 92 Affirmations That Apply Positive Quotes And Positive Words To Banish Negative Thinking by Gary Vurnum

CHARTING THE UNKNOWN

Anatomy of the Spirit by Caroline Myss

FORGIVENESS AND GRATITUDE

The Power of Positive Thinking by Norman Vincent Peale
The Tibetan Art of Positive Thinking: Skillful Thought for Successful Living by Christopher Hansard

GENERAL REFERENCES

When Things Fall Apart by Pema Chodron
Embracing The Beloved by Stephen & Ondrea Levine

Shattered

ABOUT THE AUTHOR

MARC MAISLEN has led an eclectic life. After dropping out of pre-med in college to pursue a career in dance, he performed with The American Mime Theatre in New York and went on to created original theatre/dance works with his own performing company.

He was an Artist-in-Residence at Massachusetts College of Art and taught at various universities. After leaving the East coast for the West, he became Operations Director for a K-8 school then a fundraiser for Climate Solutions in Seattle. Several years later, having survived a near-death experience and responding to his deepest calling, the Arts, Marc moved to Oregon where he currently directs, designs and performs at The Newport Performing Arts Center with his company New Visions Arts.

"Shattered..." is Maislen's first book. His second book being published simultaneously is "The Tale of Jinny Coreen." A children's book for all ages, it reflects the power of good in overcoming evil and that people can live together in harmony.

Marc lives on the Oregon Coast with his wife and two huskies and has five children and six grandchildren.

Made in the USA
Columbia, SC
24 July 2021